HORMONAL HYPNOSIS
SOME KIND OF SUPERSTAR

Series One, Episode Three

C.A. GREAGEN

Title: Hormonal Hypnosis
Some Kind of Superstar - Series One, Episode Three
Author: C.A. Greagen

Publisher: Overhead Press
Victoria, Australia
Cover Design: Greg Tuck

Connect with C. A. Greagen

Website:
www.cagreagen.com

Social Networks
Twitter: https://twitter.com/ReservoirDad
Facebook: http://www.facebook.com/ReservoirDad
Instagram: https://www.instagram.com/c.a.greagen

CONTENTS

No Touching

76:32:22

Sylvia woke me as she was getting ready for work to ask me if we had any Panadol, and after explaining how to find the key for the locked medicine box in the third drawer of the upstairs bathroom, I reach for my iPhone, pretty happy to be feeling less hung-over than I thought I would, throwing the ball to Barnaby for thirty seconds to fill his love meter, and then opening my personal Facebook page, suddenly beset upon by fear when I see a recent update by Jen which reads, "Trying to keep a positive outlook", because I still haven't heard from her since the sour ending to dinner Monday night.

Sylvia comes back into the bedroom with a glass of water just as I'm sending Jen a text asking if she and Audrey need a lift to school this morning and I spend no more than a minute, noting that the time is 6.20, giving up on hoping for the talking bubble with the little dots in it to appear, before I double press the button on my phone and bring the Facebook Pages app up. I have 3,901 Likes now and, unsurprisingly, among the many notifications is one informing me that the fan page *Doug – Exotic Dancer* mentioned me in a post.

'I can't believe how hung-over I feel,' Sylvia says, sitting on the bed with one shoe on, head in her hand, as I read some of the other notifications. I've also been mentioned by *Nude Men with Tattoos*, *Tea and Twinks Break*, and *Two Men an Hour* which I probably have Gus to thank for.

'We shouldn't have had any more to drink once we got home,' I say, opening and closing my mouth, feeling my cheeks are a bit crusty from Sylvia's full frontal assault on me. 'Why don't you just stay home? Do you really have to go in?'

'I have to fire a *lot* of people this morning,' Sylvia says. 'But I'm going to get home in time to come to school with you.'

'You're coming to the meeting about Dylan?'

'Yeah,' she says, finally getting her other shoe on. 'I want to.'

'I love you,' I say, with a teary kind of smile as I reach over to touch her back and also tap *Doug – Exotic Dancer*'s profile pic to check out his page.

'What?'

'I just really love you,' I say. 'I'm pretty nervous about this meeting.'

When I scroll down quickly to find the picture of me piggy-backing Sylvia, I pass by another photo that was posted later and so scroll back to see that it's of Doug out at a nightclub of some sort, arm in arm with another man who's wearing a tight black crop top and black jeans with a silver belt.

'Are you kidding me?' I say, thrusting the phone in front of Sylvia.

Sylvia has a look then stands up and smooth's down her skirt, reaches for her earrings on the bedside table and, as she puts them in, says, 'What did you expect? We built his expectations up all night. He must have been as horny as hell.'

After looking back at the picture, shaking my head – I mean, the possibility that he would continue on without us just never entered my mind – I'm surprised that the only way I can find to express myself is to say, 'That…*slut.*'

Sylvia laughs, puts her hand to her mouth for a moment and then, as if the thought just occurred to her, says, 'I can't believe you said he can stay here.'

'Oh, yeah,' I say, remembering the conversation on the carousel and the later conversation in the taxi, before we dropped Doug outside his agent's house, when he asked us if it was still okay to move in this week. 'Shit. But you seemed really happy about it.'

'I was drunk, Joel. And you were the one who said it was okay to begin with,' she says, opening her workbag, sliding in her MacBook Air and several files. 'And what about the ground rules?'

'We didn't make any ground rules,' I say. 'We only *talked* about making ground rules.'

'Well,' Sylvia says. 'One of the ground rules is don't involve the male sex toy you found on Craigslist in your family life. That's like 101 of *unsaid, plainly obvious to almost everybody,* ground rules.'

'Oh, there are un*said* ground rules…' I say, my neck and forehead suddenly feeling hot. 'We should probably say those unsaid ground rules out loud.'

'I'll put some thought in to them,' she says.

'We have a very large house…we have seven bedrooms,' I say, before the reality of what I've done hits me in a clear, un-inebriated way. 'Jesus, it'll be okay, won't it?' I'm scrolling through dozens of Twitter notifications to calm myself. Many of them are retweets of Doug's retweet of my *original* Tweet which was automatically Tweeted when Sylvia Instagrammed the photo of Doug and me riding seahorses together. 'Doug…doesn't seem like a *murderer* or anything.'

'Doug's nice,' Sylvia says. 'I really like him. But he comes across as a bit needy.'

'Really? He didn't seem needy to me at all.'

'You probably missed a lot of the early conversation we had about his family because you were freaking out and hiding inside your phone,' she says.

I'm about to react to the inherent snarkiness in that comment but manage to control myself by opening Candy Crush, and it's as I'm reminding myself that Sylvia is hungover and probably really stressed about sending people home to their families without jobs for the next few weeks, that I get a text from Jen, which reads, "That'd be great, Joel" and I'm just so relieved.

'Okay,' Sylvia says, ready for work, bag over her shoulder. 'Here are a few ground rules: One…no sucking cock unless I'm there with you.'

'What are you talking about?'

'You're not allowed to do anything with anyone else unless I'm there. It'd be like cheating on me. This has to be something we do together or not at all.'

'I would never…' I say pausing, genuinely confused. 'I thought we were finished with that? Haven't we *done* the cock sucking thing now?'

'Why would you even think that? You barely touched it with your lips. Silly,' Sylvia says, throwing the curtains open and turning off the light, holding her phone towards me so that I can see her stopwatch app reads, 76:45:13. 'I'm still sure you'll get the job done properly within seven days…a little over ninety-five hours left.'

'Oh my God.'

'Two…no touching yourself unless I'm with you, either. I mean, no touching at all, ever, unless I say it's okay. I want you horny and ready to go *all* the time,' she says, sitting on the bed, all smiles, eyes shining suddenly. She leans over to kiss me, rubbing her hand over the bulge

I'm trying to hide under the doona. 'Also, instead of sending me lonely old penis pictures, I want you to send me the whole package, okay? I want abs and chests and arms and faces.'

'Why?' I say, staring at the ceiling, frowning, phone quacking like a duck.

'You don't have to worry, Joel,' she says, turning my face towards her. 'Everything will work out when it all becomes more…familiar. Say good morning to Dylan for me. Tell him I'm coming to his school today.'

'Okay,' I say, watching her walk towards the door. 'Hey, what if I need to have a piss?'

She stops, shrugs, smiles. 'I guess you'll just have to sit down.'

FAMILY SUPPORT

77:47:13

In an attempt to improve my writing, I stayed in bed after Sylvia left and purchased fourteen books, using my iBook app, hoping to absorb the skills of some famous authors. But after reading 9% of The Great Gatsby, I abandoned the idea altogether because – although it does seem to be well-written – it's a totally *boring* book with no realistic sex scenes, no swearing, and not one mention of the Internet.

'Hey, Dyl,' I say, gently waking Dylan, feeling very happy with what I've achieved in the past hour despite the failed reading experiment, having showered and dressed, cleared three more levels on Candy Crush, deleted and responded to over thirty Facebook comments from last night's post, many of which have been positive, thanks mostly, I think, to the gay sites that have followed me and the hundreds of people I've been blocking.

Dylan opens his eyes, rolls from the left and to the right in a full stretch, hands above his head, cute as a button.

'Let's go. Beautiful day outside. Sun's shining, birds are chirping…' I say, opening the curtains to let the daylight in and noticing the rat-dog Diggity running around the neighbour's yard, barking like its arse is on fire. '…

annoying yap yap dogs waiting for their crushed glass and minced meat breakfast.'

'Look, Dad,' he says, hopping out of bed with a book in his hand. 'I finished it.'

'Wow,' I say, turning *Ripley's Believe It or Not* over in my hands. 'You read it from start to finish?'

Dylan nods, takes it back from me, and throws it onto the pile of books in front of his bookcase as I search for his school clothes, so annoyed that Diana's last cleaner – a young, tall, chiselled African man – has put the shorts in the wrong drawer.

'Dad,' Dylan says. 'Santana drowned on the island, and the man hung thousands of dolls to keep her happy.'

'Believe it or not!' I say, finally finding his clothes and kneeling down to help Dylan out of his pyjamas. 'Mummy and I are coming to your school today. We're going to talk to Mrs. Fox and Mrs. Brogan and the psychologist about how you can be...I don't know...*different* at school.'

'Mummy's coming?' he says.

'Yep,' I say, pulling his jumper over his school shirt, instructing him to sit down so that I can put his socks on, and then, as I'm looking for his reader bag under his bed, he jumps on top of me, starts really yanking on my neck to the point where it hurts and so I roll to the side, catching him and flipping him, moving my hands as he tries to catch them so that I can keep tickling him all over, and I'm kind of amazed by how nice this is as I listen to him laughing and squealing, screaming, 'Stop, Daddy!'. I feel like I've been missing this. It's as if it hasn't happened for a while.

'I don't *want* to be different at school,' Dylan says, a frown appearing beneath his long, straight-cut fringe while I make a half-hearted attempt to restack his bookcase, knowing that Diana will have a new young male cleaner up here this morning, anyway.

'You don't have to be the *same* as everyone,' I say, suddenly feeling nauseous, as if I'm betraying him to even be *half* siding with a freaking psychologist on this. 'You just have be a little bit different in how you behave…or something. I mean…like…just a *bit*.'

'I won't,' he says.

'You just have to sit still when the teacher asks you to, when the other kids are watching the white board.'

'No,' he says. 'I only play with Audrey.'

'You're the best reader, Dylan,' I say, spinning away from the bookcase to look right into his eyes. 'You're the best kid in the world to me, and to Mummy. We love you exactly like this.' I'm grabbing his face in my hands, kissing his head, holding him away from me. When I say, 'It's just that everyone has to be able to make *friends*. Everyone has to be part of a *community*', I'm surprised. It feels as if it's an idea that has been planted inside me by someone else.

Dylan and I are just standing there staring at each other. It's only regret that makes me let his face go. 'You don't really have to change. You're Dylan. We'll find our way through this and one day, we'll see that we were worrying about nothing…making a big deal about nothing. But do you know what we're going to do?'

'What?' he says.

'We're going to trick everyone into thinking that you *are* being different. We'll play a trick on *everyone*. I'm going to tell the teachers and the psychologist that you've changed now and then you pretend to act like the other kids, just some of the time, but we'll both know you haven't really changed at all. And do you know what I'm going to do if you can trick everyone for a whole week?'

'Buy me an iPhone?' he asks.

'Oh, I was going to buy you some new books. But okay, I'll buy you an iPhone.'

'And *then* some books?'

'Yes,' I say, hugging him from my kneeling position as he jumps up and down in my arms. 'I'll buy you books every week if we can trick the teachers and the psychologist together.'

'How many?' he asks.

'So many that we'll have to use one of the spare rooms here to build you a library. Although, do you know you can read books on iPads and iPhones now? You can have a library with every book in the world right in your pocket.'

Dylan stands back, widens his eyes, leaps into the air, and starts stomping around the room in a circle singing, 'Fucking hell, Daddy, Fucking hell, Daddy,' which really is hilarious but obviously inappropriate to many people who populate a primary school and I'm so in awe, thinking I may have stumbled across my greatest parenting moment ever, actually having to blink away tears when I say, 'Dylan, that kind of thing is *not* going to trick the psychologist' and he stops, *really* seems to think about it, and then nods.

'A man was one hundred and seven years old because he only ate skunks,' he says.

'Believe it or not!' I say, opening my Facebook Pages app. 'Let's do a selfie together.'

He runs and jumps into me with such enthusiasm that I lose my balance and fall on to my back, holding him in one arm, the phone out in front of us, and as I snap a gorgeous pic of Dylan with his face against my cheek, laughing, and me looking into the camera, also laughing, we hear Dad calling for me.

'Hell Pa!' Dylan runs down the hall and hugs him at the top of the stairs.

After I gather myself and catch up, Dad looks at me as he rocks Dylan back and forth between his titanium knees and says, 'Well?'

'Well, what?' I say, expecting nothing but strangeness from the Internet-famous Hell Pa.

To keep his question from Dylan, he makes it clear to me, by making an O-shape with his mouth and gesturing towards it several times in a row with one finger, that he's miming a blow job and then finally says out loud, 'Did you do it?'

I cannot believe the way the world turns, and I don't know whether to be amused or horrified and in the second that passes before I squeeze by them, skipping down the stairs, yelling over my shoulder, 'There's a man named Doug moving in with us this week,' I decide that it's okay to feel both of those things.

When I get into the kitchen, Diana jumps down from the bench stool, closes her interior design manual, and says, uncharacteristically, 'Hi, Joel' so that I actually freeze, moving my eyeballs only, looking around the room for the surveillance teddy, or some other kind of spying device. 'How was your night?'

'I had…a *fun* night, Diana,' I say, suddenly nervous, hearing what sounds like some excited whispering down that hall, followed by several double-handed high fives. 'I had a fun night… *Diana.*'

I'm reaching inside the kitchen cabinet for Dylan's cereal when she says, 'Dylan was just gorgeous,' and manage to turn back towards the kitchen, as if by force of magic, to make my way towards the fridge for some milk, when

I'm trapped in a bear hug, only realising it's Monica after hearing her say, 'I'm so happy for you, Joel.'

'What is everyone doing?' I say, walking forward after I'm released, collecting the milk, taking a bowl and a spoon from the drawers in the island bench. 'You're all acting crazy.'

The cereal is in the bowl and the milk is poured and the spoon goes clink against the china and I'm pushing the bowl over towards Dylan, who's sitting on his usual stool, and there's Hell Pa with his arm around Monica, and Diana leaning her hips into the bench, and as Dylan digs into his breakfast, they all just keep watching me, their smiles uncontainable, their eyes moist and happy as if they're watching a grown child of theirs being married at the altar and I can think of nothing to do, as this affection seems to be passing over from them, except to Facebook this moment.

When I raise my phone, Monica, Hell Pa, Diana, and even Dylan lean further into the Island bench pulling strange faces – Hell Pa and Monica with their fists in the air in front of them, Diana with her nose scrunched about her smile – and hold their pose for the few seconds it takes for me to focus and snap.

'I don't know what comment to write,' I say, staring at the picture for a moment.

'Just write *family*,' Hell Pa says, and after doing that, I tag in Sylvia and hit publish.

Cracks in the Asphalt

Jen's holding Audrey's booster seat and wearing a tracksuit I haven't seen her in before, a kind of fawny colour, and I stop on the road outside their house instead of pulling into the driveway, leave the car running and wait for them to walk over, still a little apprehensive about the reception I might receive after telling Greg that he wasn't fulfilling Jen sexually.

Audrey's waving both hands at us and jump-skipping with joy, and after Jen opens the door, she barrels in, saying, 'You're my boyfriend, Dylan' which makes Dylan laugh shyly and is insanely cute.

While Jen buckles Audrey into the booster seat, I watch her face in the mirror and mentally rehearse my apology, thinking I have it just about right until I notice Jen lower herself onto the front passenger seat a little gingerly and then, as she actually sits down, winces and sucks in some air.

'What happened?' I say. 'Are you okay?'

'Oh, I'm okay, alright,' she says, eyebrows raised, eyes wide, lips pursed like she's trying to communicate some news without actually saying it out loud.

'Holy shit,' I say, when I finally get it. 'Did Greg...' I pause, looking into the back seat to see Dylan and Audrey squealing and whacking at their arms like a pair of fighting kangaroos, and then lowering my voice to a whisper. 'Did Greg paddle your *arse*?'

When Jen nods, beaming, to let me know that I'm at least on the right track, I'm about to celebrate but stop to ask, 'Are you okay?' because she really does look to be in pain and it's not until she says, 'I'm *more* than okay,' that I become so overwhelmed to have done some good in the world – to have actually *helped* people. I hug her, ecstatic. 'That's just so un*real*. Oh my God. I'm so happy.'

Jen laughs, and I can tell by her expression that she feels just like I did when I was under the gaze of my family's happiness an hour ago. 'We'll have to talk about this a little later, I think,' she says, rolling her eyes towards the back seat, then laughing again.

I launch away from the curb so that the tyres spin and squeal, which is something I also *never* do, and turn up the radio full bore, taking a chance that there'll be a decent song on, drumming at the dashboard with both hands.

'Don't you just feel like everything's okay, sometimes?' I say, as we finally get out on to Boulderwood Road and hightail it towards the school. 'Like things are just the way they are? Like every day *has* to happen the way it does but that...you know...as if the universe is trying to get you all freaked out and upset…but that it's just *tricking* you – like one of those candid camera shows – so that it can jump out at you one day and say, "Hey, sucked in! It was just a joke!"'

'Yep,' Jen says, and I find myself pointing at the radio, almost involuntarily, when 'Pony' starts.

'I know a guy who can dance really well to this,' I say, jittery all of a sudden, switching the radio to another song I haven't heard of before.

'I love this song,' Jen says.

'Who is it?'

'I can't remember what it's called. It's by Drake. It's really big right now.'

By the time we reach the school, I'm certain I'm going to download this song and listen to it every chance I get, over and over and over again, until the thrill wears off, until it becomes less amazing and so boring that I never listen to it again.

We're earlier than I hoped to be, which means more time in the playground and yes, that does trigger some nerves, but I'm floating on a high right now and ready for anything.

'God,' Jen says, as I hold the door open so that the kids can jump out on the footpath. 'There's Charlotte and her cling-ons.'

Charlotte is hand in hand with Sebastian, crossing the road in front of Paul, who's standing in the middle of the children's crossing with a whistle in his mouth, clinging to the stop sign.

When he holds up his *how* hand, I hold up *my* how hand and because Charlotte's watching me without looking at Paul, she scowls and shakes her head, obviously thinking I'm waving at her – which is ridiculous because I'm actually imagining running her over with my car – before joining the righteous group of parents, who are plainly the most prestigious in the entire school.

They're all laughing, sneering at me, shaking their heads slowly, like a bunch of cats watching a pendulum, and I get this sense of a timer starting, which is counting down to the beginning of a war; Charlotte and her army against me and mine.

"@theage, @BenPobjie and @vinsurfer are Tweeting about #easter" and by the time I've looked up from that notification and closed my phone cover, Charlotte's army, in what seems to be an orchestrated move, walk around to the other side of the main building and so Jen and I follow Dylan and Audrey across the quadrangle.

My mirror sunglasses sometimes make me feel a little *rock star*, I have to admit to that, and even though I notice the people staring at me – all the women sitting on the wall-mounted bench outside the classroom, the two women looking out from the canteen, and the two dads standing, arms crossed, on the steps of the multipurpose room – I don't really care because my online audience is changing, for the better I think, and this *offline* audience is just becoming less relevant. This is confirmed when I get a Facebook notification and look to see that the gay fan page, *Guys You Wouldn't Kick Out Of Bed For Farting* has started following me.

I follow back immediately and then show Jen, who laughs outrageously, before looking up to see Mrs. Brogan picking up litter around the sand pit and I get a buzz, some real drive, and such a sense of purpose that I know without even thinking it, that I really, *really* want to be on the school council, because yes, it *will* further my potential future career in the helping professions, but also because it will be a great strategic move in the Charlotte war.

Jen follows me over, leaving Dylan and Audrey to continue running circles around the flag pole, and we get to Mrs. Brogan just as she's facing away from us, bending over the sandpit, fishing out an empty Vege Chips packet – Dylan's favourite.

After she stands up and shakes the packet free of sand, I practically shout, 'Hello, Mrs. Brogan' to get her attention, so that she yips like a kicked dog and turns, pulling on her skirt self-consciously.

'Hello,' she says. 'I was looking for you.'

'I was just wondering if you've had a chance to talk to the members of the school council. I'm still very keen to accept your invitation to join.'

'Well, Joel,' she says, suddenly so *principal* in her expression. 'We voted on it, and unfortunately—'

'I can make a difference. I have some great ideas for fundraising.'

'We've already filled the position,' she says, pausing. 'But maybe you can try again next year?'

'The bike sheds really need a coat of paint…and there are large cracks in the asphalt, in the quadrangle,' I say, desperately, overwhelmed by a sense of loss that I can only attribute to the real desire to be on the council, or the need to gain an upper hand on Charlotte, or the fact that I'm sleep-deprived and more hungover from last night than I realise. 'You said you wanted another *dad* on the council.'

'We found another dad.

'Who?' I ask, genuinely surprised.

'Simeon,' she says.

'Simeon?' I say, getting all goady. 'What's a Simeon?'

'That's Simeon over there,' she says, pointing between the administration building and the grade 5/6s classroom to a circular bench with a tree in the middle where Charlotte and her cronies – all cat heads staring at us – are sitting, and in amongst them is that single short, unspoken bearded man who's always there but who becomes invisible to you, kind of like a wart on your best friend's neck.

'Is *that* Simeon?' I say, pointing. 'Is Simeon *that* man right there? That man who always stands behind Charlotte agreeing with her…in a nonverbal way?'

'Joel—'

'He's just an…an un-uttering…puppet. I mean…I've never even seen him with a kid. Does he have one?'

Mrs. Brogan is looking at me, slack-jawed, and I know I should really cut my losses here and move on – I actually *hate* councils of *any* sort – but last night, I was on my knees in a haunted castle with an exotic dancer's dick on my lips. An exotic dancer so amazingly hot and so great at dancing that every council-appointed mum in the *world* would have swapped places with me in a second and, I don't know, I somehow feel stronger because of it; I feel like I'm in possession of a unique experience that elevates me in a way, that gives me more clout, more *flair*, that means I should stand my ground, that means I shouldn't let anyone push me around. And it's as I'm getting an *emotional* rise – feeling like I could actually break down and cry with happiness – that a piece of the puzzle falls into place with me and, emboldened to the point of *sniff*-laughing to cover the horror of what I'm about to ask, I say, 'Is Charlotte on the council, as well?'

'Charlotte's head of fundraising,' Mrs. Brogan says, folding her arms. 'She's very creative.'

'Well, Mrs. Brogan,' I say, pushing my sunglasses farther up the bridge of my nose, flipping my phone cover open, closing it again, stepping backwards and then forwards. 'You've just filled two positions on the school council with one ventriloquist act.'

I look to Jen for support and receive it in the form of an excellently timed eye-roll. 'Jen, tell Mrs. Brogan about Sebastian's reader diary,' I say, actually folding my arms.

'I…won't,' Jen says, looking down at the ground suddenly, glancing at me out of the corner of her eyes, seemingly terrified of saying *anything* in front of Mrs. Brogan.

'She writes these ridiculous descriptions about the books he reads,' I say, speaking for Jen. 'And she colours in all the columns and boxes, and it's all so sickly sweet when she talks at school meetings and so over-the-top that it's obvious she's trying to make everyone think she's some super…great…self-sacrificing parent when the truth that everyone can see…is that she's using her kid to elevate her social standing…kind of like Munchausen syn—'

'Joel!' she says, more forcefully this time. 'This isn't appropriate, and this is exactly why we voted against you joining the council.'

'What do you mean?' I say, looking over my shoulder at Charlotte's army because I can smell the smugness hovering around them like a thick dark cloud of poisonous, foetus-deforming dust. I just want to beat them so *much*, and there's a kind of thrill in the way I'm losing myself here.

Mrs. Brogan scans the school yard, steps closer to me, and then in a lower tone, says, 'You can live however you want, and *behave* however you want in your own home, but you cannot share disgusting pictures and write pornographic blog posts referring to a member of our school council as a bitch. You cannot threaten to run over a parent at this school and expect to become a member of its council.'

'I'm not really such a great writer,' I say, as a kind of defence. 'What's in my head doesn't often come out the way I mean it.'

'So what *did* you mean by saying that?' she asks. 'What did you *mean*, Joel, when you attacked a member of our school community like that?'

'That you shouldn't let...people push you around,' I say, searching for the right words. 'That you shouldn't let them push you around like that.'

The music stops and the bell sounds and I'm surprised to detect a level of snarkiness in Mrs. Brogan that I hadn't seen before. She actually looks pleased with herself, and it strikes me that her expression – smiling on one side of her mouth, simmering intent behind her piercing eyes, the complete *arsehole* emoticon – is exactly how I picture the expressions of the people who leave "fucking faggot" comments on my Facebook page.

'You had such a nice little blog,' she says, as a way of finishing the conversation. 'You and Hell Pa could have really been of service to the school by sharing our sausage sizzles on your Facebook page and promoting our chocolate drives to your Twitter followers. We were looking forward to you joining the council. We thought you'd really fit in. But then…I have no idea what happened to you. You and Hell Pa have just become another form of *smut* on the Internet.'

'You said you loved Hell Pa.'

'He posts so many pictures of nudity that I've had to unfollow him on Instagram,' she says. 'Maybe you should suggest he paint a landscape, or a bowl of fruit, like a *real* artist.'

The sound of my temples pulsing, which started as soon as I heard 'nice little blog', lingers on even as my distracting anger is offset by how hilarious she sounded saying 'sausage sizzle' and 'chocolate drive', and I want to come up with something amazing to say to defend Dad but I find myself just staring at her, as if we're from different cultures and simply not capable of communicating through our differences. If I have rebelliousness towards *anything*, it's towards *rigidity*, and there's rigidity right there, standing before me in human form.

It's just as Mrs. Brogan is passing me that she lifts her gaze towards the Charlottes and smiles and I'm certain, without looking, that they're all smiling back at her, in the way that people do when they *are* from the same culture.

And suddenly, I just don't care; I'm Doug jumping backwards over a chair at The Dragon Fly, Diana throwing away expensive paintings and hiring sexy Twink cleaners, Sylvia showing my cock pics to the women at work, Monica moving into an art studio and posing nude for an old man, Dad transforming from a retired suicidal banker into Hell Pa *the artist* within the span of one night, and Dylan, who swears, rebels, sleeps with hardback books, and loves me all at the same time.

'I have the greatest fundraising idea, Mrs. Brogan.'

'And what's that, Joel?'

After what feels like minutes of suspended animation, I blurt out, 'Hell Pa's going to have an art exhibition. It will be so popular it'll make more for the school in one night than Charlotte could make with a *year's* worth of sausage sizzles.'

Mrs. Brogan laughs and becomes a member of the pendulum-following cat-heads and says something like *I don't think that will pass by council for approval* but I don't care because I've dug my heels in and after Jen says, 'The kids are going in,' we head over to the entrance to the prep classroom and catch Dylan and Audrey, last in line as usual, before they make it inside.

'New iPhone, Dad?' Dylan whispers, when I bend down to kiss his head.

'What are you going to do?' I whisper back.

'Trick everyone,' he says.

'Yesssss,' I say.

'We'll see you this afternoon for the meeting?' Mrs. Fox says.

'We'll see you this afternoon for the meeting,' I say.

Multi-Mum

79:25:19

I tried to convince Jen that her brother is *not* autistic because after holding his hand up as we passed by on the way to the car, I'm pretty certain I saw him push his tongue into his left cheek while pumping his right hand towards his mouth a few times, basically calling me a cocksucker, but Jen – after rabbiting on about his amazing sense of humour – educates me on the autistic *spectrum*, and tells me that we all have autism, just to varying degrees, which I find very hard to believe.

On the way to Jen's house, I gave her my phone and asked her to find that new Drake song and it took a bit of messing around until she finally found it, and then a bit more time before I was able to dictate my iTunes password – !dyldylanddyl37:) – to her effectively, so we really didn't get the chance to talk about the story behind her abused buttocks, as I'd hoped. When she asked me to come in for a coffee, I turned the car off and decided my plan to go to the gym could be put off for an hour or so. And it was only then that I felt this pure exhaustion.

'Are you okay?' Jen asks, as she opens the front door and I follow her into the house.

'I think I'm actually a little freaked out. I wasn't expecting that kind of confrontation.'

'You were so amazing,' Jen says, glazed over for a moment. 'I could never confront people like that.'

'Sometimes,' I say, with effort; the raw energy charging through me in the schoolyard seems to have been depleted. 'I get this…*high*…and I manage to climb out of myself somehow…to behave with less…restriction.'

At first, I'm surprised to see that Jen's house is so cluttered. Just in the lounge room, dining area, and kitchen, which are all basically the one space in the shape of a block letter U, there are several wooden cabinets and bookshelves overflowing with books and magazines and photos, as well as various trinkets including many, *many* fairy figurines.

The couch is oversized and crammed into the lounge area, piled with cushions that don't really match its brown vinyl. The chairs take up most of the dining area, to the point where it would be impossible to walk without moving one chair at a time, and I'm thinking it would be really great for Diana to flex some of her interior redesigning *madness* over here, when I notice that space under the kitchen bench – where you'd normally have some stools – is taken up by two clothes horses, one of which is overloaded with Jen's identically designed and sized, *differently* coloured tracksuits.

The kitchen bench seems ordered and clean but is overflowing with electrical appliances, a bread box, notepads and pens, glass containers filled with sugar, coffee, cereal, and pasta and it's only when I become removed from the focus on my own exhaustion – so fascinated by the utter lack of space – that I realise the issue is not that Jen and Greg have so many possessions – Sylvia and I own a lot more *things* – it's that their house is so incredibly small. We could fit Jen's entire lounge, dining, and kitchen area inside our bedroom. Sylvia and I are only able to present ourselves as orderly and uncluttered because of the space available to us inside the monstrosity. The house we own casts a shadow over me and gives me a chill. I feel like an arsehole.

'I'm sorry,' Jen says, reaching in between a blender and a toaster and under a wall-mounted cupboard to turn on a kettle.

'Don't be silly,' I say, a little desperately. 'You have a really *nice* house.'

Jen takes a quick glance and smiles a little before returning her focus to filling the kettle. 'I mean, I'm sorry for not sticking up for you in front of Mrs. Brogan when you asked about Charlotte.'

'Oh,' I say, mortified that I just implied some insecurity on Jen's part, or most likely, some assumed *privilege* on my part, but lacking the energy to even cringe. 'I'm probably not seeing this clearly, but it really feels like they're out to get me.'

'It's just because you're not like everyone else,' she says, with a shrug, as if she's no stranger to this kind of tension. 'So many people at the school hate Charlotte already. I hear them talking about her. And no one likes

Mrs. Brogan. She's an import from Brighton where the mums wear more makeup and nicer clothes and have cleaners and nannies and heaps of time to do more for the school. She doesn't *get* people like us. But everyone just acts so nice around her…and some of the mums who hate Charlotte act like total fan girls whenever she's actually around.'

'I don't *hate* Charlotte,' I say. 'I'd never admit *that*.'

'You're strange like that, though,' Jen says, handing me a coffee. 'You just seem to move on. I was so angry after she attacked you on her Facebook page.'

'She what?'

'That whole campaign she did last Saturday. When she told everyone you were a pervert and that you threatened to kill her and…how she wrote an email to that horrible current affairs program, *The Daily Events*.'

'She what?'

'It was great how some people stuck up for you.' As she's stirring sugar into her coffee, I can see it dawning on her that I have no idea what she's talking about. 'You didn't see what Charlotte said about you? On her *Multi-Mum* Facebook page?'

'Charlotte is *Multi-Mum*?' I say, kind of whisper-shrieking, as if there are two hands around my throat, choking me. 'I'd chosen to hide all her posts from my feed…'

'I know,' Jen says, walking to the kitchen table. 'She's just a pure hate read for me. All her articles on how to brighten your bathroom or throw a dinner party or pick the perfect flower arrangement.' Jen stops to lower herself slowly into the kitchen chair, wincing and leaning into the table to shift the weight off the meatier part of her buttocks. 'And how about those photos of her and Sebastian…there's one every day of them throwing a Frisbee or picking daisies or just looking into each other's eyes. And the school lunches she makes… cucumber pieces cut into the letter S and the…*I love you* pastry messages on her homemade vegetarian pasties. I just want to throw a vegemite sandwich at her.'

'She has like…a *lot* of Facebook Likers,' I say, phone open, typing *Multi-Mum* into the search box on my personal Facebook page.

'One hundred and eighteen thousand,' Jen says.

'One hundred and *twenty* thousand now,' I say, as I'm scrolling through two days' worth of her posts – about twelve in total – until I'm stunned to see that she's shared my blog banner and after holding it up to show Jen, as if she hadn't already seen it, I start reading the post titled 'Evil in Our School'.

"First a massive thank you. This community has been such an amazing support to me over the past three years. I consider you more supportive to me than my own family. After starting my little page, I had no idea of the sisterhood that I would find. I was lost, struggling as a single mum, wondering how I was going to get by after my husband left me, and if it wasn't for the Multi-Mum community that took me under its wing, I might still be addicted to anti-depressants.

I am now not addicted to anti-depressants and I make a really great income through my blog. I am a member of the school council and Sebastian is thriving. I'm so proud of him. Even though he has done it all himself, it really is thanks mostly to me, for rising above the worst that life could have thrown at me, and that means it's also thanks to you, my followers. I really hope that I have given as much back to you as you've given to me in the form of better ways to decorate your house, how to make you child thrive, creating better doilies for your tissue boxes and toilet rolls, and basically improving as a homemaker. But most importantly, I hope I've improved you as a mum.

The reason I am calling on you now is that there is a father, whose son (I won't name, he seems to have a disability, and it's not his fault anyway) goes to school with Sebastian. This father, if you can actually call him that, has the Facebook page *D-D-Dad?* (Ironical?) which I won't tag in because I don't want to further its filth and he has recently been posting pictures of penises, and describing those penises.

And even more disturbing was that he threatened to kill me in his last blog post, which you can read here, because I was courageous enough to call him what he is in the playground. A pervert.

Don't get me wrong, I am not anti-gay. I am always sharing posts about gay rights and marriage equality even though I am morally dead against it. I just think that there's a time and a place to be THAT gay and it's not on Facebook in the twentieth century. Gay sex belongs in the home. Otherwise, you're a pervert. Pretty simple.

I have written to *The Daily Events* to expose this man. And so far, they have been pretty interested in following it up. We've had several emails, and they say they love my page.

And this is how I am calling on the Multi-Mum community who not only share my values but also know that if we don't stand up against smut and filth and protect our children, then who will?

Please spread this message. Please Like it and Share it. Tag in all your friends and ask them to boycott *D-D-Dad?* He actually wants to join our school council. Can you believe that? It makes me shiver. I am so tired of privileged white men mansplaining courageous women out of important positions. Thank you for your support. Kisses for all, Multi-Mum."

The first thing that strikes me as I'm reading this ruinous post is that Charlotte is clearly an amazing writer, and even though I'm already *burning* to write something to defend myself, I am, at this moment, so certain she'll use her superior academic skill to pull apart any blog post I write in response to hers, that I actually just give in.

'Okay, then. I actually do hate Charlotte now,' I say to Jen. 'In the past week, I've been called a fucking faggot dozens of times, I've been told I promote smut on the Internet, I've been publicly…humiliated really…by people who don't know me at all, and now a post calling me a pervert, written by—'

'That bitch?' Jen suggests.

'…has been shared one thousand, three hundred and twenty-three times. But fuck it. This happened two days ago, and two days ago is like a lifetime ago in social media.'

'It really is,' Jen says.

'And I know, from personal experience,' I say, looking through some of the comments under the post, most of which are sharing in Charlotte's faux-outrage, many just saying something like, "Disgusting. Shared". 'That Charlotte is not really so outraged by what I did. She's not trying to "protect our children". She's just trying to get more Likes. That's what all this is about. And…'

Jen says something else supportive which I don't catch because I get a notification that a person I follow on

Twitter; *@JodieMcClelland*, who I don't actually know, has just opened an Instagram account.

'And it was while all this *mania* was happening – while Charlotte was checking her Facebook page every two minutes last night, probably freaking out that the Likes and the Shares were slowing down on her post…probably considering sponsoring it because it had such great *organic* reach – that I was having a great time with Sylvia. I was having a…really *great* time…with Sylvia.'

When I stop talking, I become aware of the tension in my jaw and neck and my abs are so tense, they're vibrating a little, restricting my breathing, and I look from my phone to Jen, caught off guard with how she's looking at me.

At first, I'm not quite sure why it makes me think of myself standing in front of the prep classroom on Dylan's first day of school, but then I realise it's because her expression – the pensive, smiling emoticon – reminds me of how I was feeling then: as Dylan walked through the school classroom and found his place on the floor in front of the bookcase, I was remembering my own school experience, aware that he was entering a world that might not quite fit with him, that might cause him more suffering than joy, hoping that he might actually find his place but knowing that there was nothing I could really do about it.

'I hate Charlotte,' I say, checking my phone because I thought I heard Barnaby whimpering but opening the

Virtual Dog app to see that all his meters are full and that he's panting at me, spinning around, wagging his tail, happy.

Jen laughs, holds her fists up. 'We can bitch about her together.'

'Throughout this whole disaster,' I say. 'There's been this thing happening where masses of people are Un-Liking me, abusing me so that I ban them, or permanently hiding all my posts. But then right now, I have more followers than I ever have, I'm getting even *more* comments, more Shares, and more supportive messages. It's like I'm finding out who my *real* friends are.'

'Charlotte is just a big faker,' Jen says. 'She'd have no idea who actually likes her. Offline or online.'

'I'm just going to forget all about her,' I say, flipping the cover on my phone, scrolling through her Facebook page. 'Why waste my time. I'm so wound up all the time.'

'She's really not worth it.'

'Oh my God,' I say, holding my phone towards Jen again. 'She's organised a sausage sizzle for the school this Sunday.'

'Joel, you can sit down if you want.'

I am suddenly aware of myself as a forever reforming tsunami, set in motion by a force I can't quite see, or pinpoint, set in motion by a force that draws me back, *way* back – a long, long way – before it drives me forwards *raging,* charging over the people who have gathered on the exposed ocean floor to see the colourful, jagged coral and the stunned, suffocating sea life.

'We have to have Hell Pa's exhibition on the same day,' I say, reaching for the chair.

'Oh, you're really going to do that?'

'I promised Mrs. Brogan I'd raise money,' I say, pulling the chair out slowly, noting how poorly the sausage sizzle post has performed, receiving only 26 Likes, 2 comments, and *no* Shares. 'To paint the bike sheds and…fix the asphalt.'

'It's going to be hard to organise it in time,' Jen says.

'We should synchronise our Google Calendars,' I say, sitting down without looking up from my phone and so surprised to feel a short sharp pain in my right bum cheek that I actually throw my phone on the table as I jump back to an upright position.

'I'm sorry!' Jen says, throwing her phone next to mine when she sees me holding a broken wooden spoon and a snapped studded dog collar. 'I thought I'd put those away.'

'I'm okay,' I say. 'Are these what I think they are?'

Jen giggles into her hand and avoids my eyes. 'Last night…I've never felt so—'

'Me, either,' I say, promising myself I'll listen to her without looking at my phone or getting distracted by my internal world, which is constantly in flux and never certain. 'I really thought you were going to get a divorce. I really thought I'd ruined your life.'

'I thought you had, as well,' she says, suddenly so animated. 'God, Greg was so angry that I'd told you about our sex life. When we got home and wouldn't talk to me, but then he came into our bedroom where I'd been playing Candy Crush — I always do that when I'm depressed — for almost the entire day and started crying. We had the best talk because…he hates his job. He wanted to be a pro wrestler when we first started going out and now, he's just collecting drinks and saying 'legs eleven' every day and because he doesn't really have many friends — he doesn't have Facebook or anything — he just feels like a failure. He doesn't feel like he's accomplished anything.'

'I get that,' I say.

'Yeah,' Jen says, hands flying, eyes wide, her biggest smile. 'And we just realised we were depressed. We *both* were. And then I remembered your post and read it to him and we talked about that and about how *amazing* it was that even people like you and Sylvia could feel just like we did…so far away from each other. And that even people like you and Sylvia had to try different things.'

'Wow,' I say.

'And the biggest thing, something that I just *never* would have thought of, is that…maybe…it's not…that you've stopped having sex because your relationship is falling apart, but—'

'That your relationship is falling apart because you're not having sex,' I say, and suddenly, I'm mirroring her eyeballs, not crying, not even allowing my eyes to water and…*fuck* Charlotte.

'We were looking up different sites and learning about BDSM and we had some JB cans and we tried all these different things. Really basic things mostly, like spanking and paddling and verbal abuse and oh my *God…*'

I am in such suspense as I wait for Jen to pull herself out of her sudden inwardness, as I wait for the glaze in her eyes to disappear, that I find myself wishing she was a touch screen, so that I could swipe past this low impact scene to the point where she starts talking again.

'And the sex was…not quite everything I've ever dreamed about…but the most amazing sex I've ever had. Greg really got into it. I mean, he *really* got in to it, to the point where he stopped asking me if I was okay and just relied on me using the safe word. And that's how the collar got broken,' she says, shifting the hood on her tracksuit top to show me a long, thin abrasion on her neck. 'And that's why my bum's so sore. He was *really* paddling me. When the wooden spoon broke on my arse, he made me say sorry for breaking it and told me he was going to punish me. And then he was…the man I've been imagining for so long. He just let go. He pulled me to my knees by my collar and started fucking…' Jen slaps a hand over her mouth and focuses in on me as if she's just realised I was there. 'He was screaming at me, asking me if I was going to take my punishment, telling me to say "Yes, Master Greg." And I kept saying it over and over until I had an orgasm and – I don't know if he meant this – he pulled on my collar tighter and tighter until I couldn't talk or breath and then it snapped and I just felt like I was floating, like I was under a spell or something.'

'Hypnotised and obedient,' I say.

'I just so…I want to have it again.'

I'm not horny listening to this story, well, not any more than usual; I am just *enthralled* and even though my iPhone and Jen's iPhone are both sounding out and vibrating notifications at such regular intervals, reminding me of two flies buzzing around a BBQ trying to mate with each other, I am able to resist the urge to grab mine.

I'm just so happy for Jen right now. I know what it feels like to reconnect like this and yes, my first thought is to announce this wonderful event on Facebook, to celebrate, but of course, it would be wrong to share someone else's story when it's of such a personal nature, and it's as I'm wondering what I can do – perhaps get her a present, a gift voucher or an iTunes card or something – that Jen shivers a little and continues.

'This morning, Greg woke me up before he went to

work. He brought me a coffee and had gotten Audrey ready for school. And then he showed me these websites that had tips on how to care for yourself after a BDSM session. He's going to buy me some ointments before he comes home and tonight, he's going to look after me and…he was so sweet and…I just haven't stopped thinking about him.'

Jen wipes her eyes as she breathes in deeply and then breathes out, her hands falling to the table and so I take the chance, when she shifts the momentum by giggling, to flip the cover on my iPhone which, it seems, gives Jen the permission to do the same thing and some minutes pass by as we're tapping and swiping away silently.

I Like several posts on my personal Facebook page, respond to a notification informing me that a man named Brian Johnson is celebrating his birthday today by writing "Happy Birthday" on his wall, and save a photo of a muscular naked man with a hard cock, making sure his whole body is visible as Sylvia requested, aware that I am finding it impossible to select a photo that includes a male *face*.

A notification from Jen's phone is the thing that causes me to look up, and when I see her gasp and laugh and slap her hand to her mouth again, I realise I'm feeling like I've let Sylvia down.

'Look.' Jen's holding her phone out so that I can see a text from Greg which reads, "How's my little slut going?"

Despite myself, I gasp as well, rebounding as usual, from one emotional stupor to the other, and am surprised to let this truth escape me. 'It's so great that Greg's done all this for you. I didn't go through with the thing Sylvia wanted me to do. I couldn't *quite* go through with it.'

'Baby steps,' Jen says, tapping into her phone. 'Greg still hasn't suspended me from the ceiling yet.'

We're both laughing and flipping the covers on our phones at the same time as I look around at the tiny space this family inhabits and think of Diana and then Doug and then Gus. 'I better go,' I say. 'I was going to go to the gym but I'm not sure…'

Jen reaches out and grasps my phoneless hand and in a kind of verbal *sprint* says, 'I've never had a friend like you,' and I'm about to repeat that back to her, because it's true, but I stop myself for some reason; because of squeamishness or uncertainty or because something was clamped shut inside me a long time ago, I'm just not sure what it is.

'I'm learning about myself just like you, Jen. I mean, I don't want to be paddled or collared or suspended from the ceiling…I don't think…but I am more aware of how I'm made now. There's this euphoria or this kind of…unthinking *happiness* when I'm treated dismissively—'

'You *are* strange,' she says, cutting me off as I stand up, push the chair in, squeeze between the clothes horse and the table, 'Some of the mums at school just think you're plain weird. But before you stop blogging, you should think about people like me and Greg, not people like Charlotte. Your blog really helps people.'

'Shut *up*,' I whisper, moved, getting more practiced at *not* crying, making my way to the door, pretending to look at some fairy trinkets in the bookcase so Jen has time to stand up, wince, and catch up to me.

When she hugs me at the door, I realise a pattern has been set in motion – Jen and I are *huggers* now. 'What level are you up to on Candy Crush?' I ask.

'Nine hundred and forty-three,' she says, laughing, and then. 'Oh, I forgot to tell you.'

I hear a whimper, and Jen's holding her phone up. 'We got a dog, as well. This is Ekko.'

'So it was Ekko whimpering before,' I say, noting his health meters, putting my mirror sunglasses on. 'You should get him into a bath really quickly and blow-dry his coat – you can buy a blow-dryer for a dollar ten if you haven't earned one already. And if you want to feed him in a way that keeps him satiated the longest, you should give him a leg of ham.'

'Okay.'

'Also,' I say, tuning back just as I'm descending the steps on the front porch. 'If you teach Ekko to perform a backwards somersault…and it *does* take a bit of time…you'll earn a woollen blanket for his kennel, which maintains his health and love meters even if you happen to neglect him for a few days.'

"Being Yourself"

82:49:10

After I'd casually told Diana, Hell Pa, and Monica that I had a personal vendetta against a mother at Dylan's school – the Internet-famous *Multi-Mum* – who I *actually* hated for defaming me on the Internet, and that I was going to enact my sweet revenge by going head to head with her in a fundraising battle, pitting her heavily backed *clichéd* sausage sizzle against the as yet unannounced *inaugural* exhibition of Hell Pa's art, in an actual art *gallery*, it was as if I'd cracked a magical whip in the air and rained cocaine dust down on their placid little heads and this entire day has been both exhilarating and frustrating.

As I'm reaching the end of my workout, getting some squat tips from Gus, the time to meet with Mrs. Brogan and Mrs. Fox and the psychologist growing nearer and nearer, I'm full of beans despite drinking last night and despite the trauma of *Multi-Mum*'s post.

'Is that your phone *again*?' Gus asks, as I rack the bar after another killer set and lean over to pick it up from beside the squat rack.

'I never usually get this many texts,' I say, opening a text from Diana to see a picture of a single story building, the fourth possible art gallery venue she's sent me in the past two hours. 'They're all so excited about the exhibition.'

'It sounds like it's going to be a heap of fun,' Gus says, wiping his face with the towel hanging around his neck and then discarding it to the floor, loading the bar on to his back, and starting his set.

'It's not that I want to humiliate *Multi-Mum* so much,' I say, as I stand behind Gus, my hands just below his armpits, squatting up and down with him in unison, spotting as he taught me. 'It's that I can raise some money for Dylan's school and you know…do something of value.'

Gus stops at the top of the squat to groan out, 'Well, you've always been keen to help people,' before taking a deep breath and squatting down again. Using the technique cues he's taught me, I look into his eyes in the mirror to say, 'Tight back, tight back,' feeling useful when he retracts his shoulders and grits his teeth. His next several reps look fast and solid.

The weight is racked, and a fist-bump later, I swipe away an Instagram notification informing me that *@strongwomanau* has started following me, to show Gus the dozen photos Hell Pa has texted me of the paintings he wants to include in the exhibition.

'Wow,' he says. 'He's really into breasts and bums and—'

'Vaginas…yeah,' I say, apologetically. 'Dad only has one live model. He really should have more. In fact, I'll text him that right now and suggest that he try for more *variety* in his work.' After sending the text and getting back under the bar for another set, I say, 'Dad has about twenty finished paintings. But if he works hard and takes some risks, he should have about thirty by Saturday.'

'Hey,' Gus says, 'Less talking, more squatting.'

After performing one squat of the ten Gus wants me to do, I pause again. 'But I really have no idea about how many paintings are required for an art exhibition. Diana told me that having less paintings, so that there is more wall space, is actually a technique used to bring an intense focus to each one, and that it's been proven that—'

'Shut up and squat!' Gus says, pausing and replacing his expression of frustration with a friendly smile to nod at a woman, saying, 'Hi, Steph' as she walks past us and up the steps to the spinning class.

'It's been proven,' I say, after performing another repetition and pausing again. 'That paintings will actually sell for more money if they're not in an overcrowded gallery.'

Gus is screaming technique cues – knees out, drive the hips forward, chest up – that sort of thing, and I've noticed that there are three men sitting on the bench beside our squat rack – really big dudes wearing the smallest items of clothing – obviously waiting for us to finish, and in the time it's taken me to perform another four reps, six in total, my phone has quacked twice and I've filled Gus in on a heap of the exhibition backstory. I'm just about totally out of breath. 'Diana's appointed herself manager and…consultant and…oh, God…she's already out and about…researching venues.'

'Eyes forward!'

'And Dad…' I say, taking a deep breath, squatting, standing up again, pausing '…is like a little kid. It's like his dream come true.'

'Squeeze the bar!'

Another text and one of the guys next to us leans forward onto his knees, shaking his head, and I wasn't even sure if I was going to get this rep, it took such a long time to just stand back up. 'I'm going to create a Facebook Event for it today…so I can…oh, fuck…begin to build some momentum.'

'Two more reps,' Gus screams, and I can see by looking at his reflection in the mirror that he's feeling pressured and when I shift my vision to look at the three big guys, one of them in particular draws my attention because he's bald and insanely muscular and reminds me of the dominant man in the website Jen showed me in the car on Monday. He catches my eyes and sneers and then lifts his pre-workout drink to his lips without losing eye contact before realising that the bottle is empty. To save face, he crushes it in his hand and growls a little.

'Let's focus,' Gus says. 'Focus, Joel. Come on, man.'

The pressure inside my head as I perform my final rep is enough to make me think I'll lose an eyeball right at the bottom of the squat, and when I look at myself in the mirror, my face almost purple, my head seemingly swelled by the rise in blood pressure, I am aware of being in that different headspace again. I feel like I've been in and out of it all day.

After completing only one more rep and racking the bar, I turn to the biggest of the three muscular guys and say, 'Your drink was already finished,' more loudly than I'd anticipated. 'You thought you had some left when you tried to intimidate me by sipping from it like the Incredible Hulk, but it completely ruined your dramatic moment, didn't it? You couldn't even rescue yourself from humiliation by crushing the empty bottle in your hand because, well, the bottle is *plastic*. It's a bottle that a *baby* could crush.'

'Joel!' Gus says, dragging me away to the other side of the squat rack just as the guy stands up and throws the plastic bottle to the floor behind him.

I swipe away an Instagram notification informing me that my Facebook friend *Jess Shute* has joined Instagram as *@shutejess* to open Hell Pa's reply to my last text, and in the second it takes for it to open, I look up to see that Gus is speaking very quietly with his back to me.

The three guys are nodding in a sympathetic way and there is an awareness inside me that I confronted them despite being very scared – my hands are shaking – and I can only put this down to the events of this past week: I am getting more practiced at absorbing abuse and intimidation.

Dad has sent me a picture of a naked young man who's smiling and giving the 'thumbs up' towards the camera, and even through Monica's photo-bombing from the side, partially obscuring him, I recognise him as Diana's cleaner for the day because he passed by me in the hall with a load of washing when I got home this morning and said 'G'day' in a thick accent. Dad's text reads, "This is Bon. He's an accounting student from Nepal. Diana and I had this great idea to do a series of paintings for one wall of the gallery called Nude Male Cleaners from Around the World."

I text "Go with it" as Gus gets back under the bar. 'Joel. Fucking *focus*. Last set.'

'It really seems to be coming together,' I say, as I squat up and down behind Gus, arms out, for ten very fast reps. 'It's crazy that I only had this idea this morning but already, we have this real…direction. We just have to hope for a great venue, I think. Diana's followed *Multi-Mum*'s page and has the address for the sausage sizzle, which is in the Archie Benson Reserve near that new children's park, so if we can manage to get as close to that as possible, we should be able to compete with her…maybe even steal some of her audience, anyway. One of the reasons I really wanted to come to the gym today, despite being really fatigued from drinking last night was to…well, fill you in on everything that's happening and then to ask you…if you wouldn't mind bouncing for us…if you'd be security for the exhibition.'

Gus racks the bar grabs his towel and water bottle, says, 'Thanks, fellas,' to the three muscular guys, and signals for me to follow him to the lockers by the exit, and I'm a bit bemused as I collect my phone, towel, and mirror sunglasses when one of them says, 'Good squatting, buddy' and slaps me on the back, as if we actually *are* buddies. When I look up to the aerobics area, I see the woman Gus spoke to earlier, Steph, riding a stationary bike, waving at me through the floor-to-ceiling windows.

Gus collects his bag and leads me out the sliding doors, down the ramp, out on to the footpath. We're walking towards our cars without a word being spoken and I'm all out of buzz, thinking Gus is completely over me, and I'm sinking right there in the open air when Gus stops beside his car. 'What was going on with you today, Joel? You were so unfocused. You have to be more aware of people around you. Those guys back there aren't bad guys. They were just frustrated because you were fussing around on your phone and talking during sets. Not everyone has hours of the day to themselves.'

'I just…I'll put my iPhone on silent when I'm at the gym from now on.'

'That's a good idea,' Gus says, his car beeping open behind him.

'Don't worry about the bouncing thing,' I say, clearing my throat, putting my mirror sunglasses on to hide away and to give Gus the chance to see how ripped he looks in the natural light. 'We can just hire someone.'

'You *can* be a little self-centred and frustrating sometimes,' Gus says, and I'm pleased to see that he turns to the right a little, angling his triceps, looking at his own reflection. 'But you're genuine. You really do care about people. I had a D&M with Craig after talking to you last week and we've come to an agreement…and beside all that, you're the most entertaining guy I have ever met.' Gus stops to laugh and then puts on his own sunglasses. 'You just don't know how *not* to be real, do you? You're the real Joel, like, *all* the time, no matter what's going on. I wouldn't miss it for anything. Consider me your Kevin Costner. I'll be your bodyguard.'

I hold out my fist, receive a fist-bump that lingers longer than usual, and say, 'Thanks Gus, I really appreciate it', just hanging there as he gets in the driver's seat and winds down the windows. After he pulls away from the curb, with Whitney Houston playing loud, I hold my fist out again, in case he's looking at me in the rear vision mirror, struck by these two thoughts – "Isn't it just a cliché that gay people like Whitney Houston?" and "Why can't I be as certain as Gus, about who the real Joel is?"

A ROUGH LANDING

85:03:32

It's 2.50pm and I've been sitting outside the school in the car since 2.30 and even though I'm nervous as hell about the meeting, I've managed to create an event on Facebook for Hell Pa's Art Exhibition which I think reads pretty well – although I'll check in with Sylvia on that. All I need before I can make the event live is the address of the venue. Then I'll invite as many people as I can, share it on all my social media platforms, even include it on the front page of my blog with a timer counting down to 2pm Sunday.

I'm watching the immovable Paul who's on the curb facing the children's crossing, holding his stop sign, as I'm talking to Sylvia. She's had to spend more time with recently fired people than she'd hoped and is hightailing it over here as fast as possible.

I've filled her in on everything that's happened today and I can tell, just from the tone of her voice, that she's angry with *Multi-Mum* and that she's angry with Mrs. Brogan and that she's just angry in *general*, but I feel a little better after talking to her and I'm just so happy and so relieved that we're meeting with the psychologist together.

Despite the lingering nerves, the sun is so warm through the windscreen that – even with the cool breeze coming through the open window – I'm struggling to stay awake and I actually zone out, miss some of Sylvia's ranting, my head dropping, my eyes mostly closed until she says, 'Okay, I'll see you in about fifteen minutes' and hangs up.

To stay awake, I check *Multi-Mum*'s Facebook page and read through some of the more defamatory comments about me and then, on a whim, still feeling just a little bit goady, I go back to the first of the 846 comments and start Liking them all as *D-D-Dad?* But then, after liking about 200 comments, I start drifting off again and so decide to write my own Facebook update – "Some people are so insecure and have no life and think that they can just pull people down to make themselves taller. And if you know who I'm talking about – or even if you don't – stay tuned because I am planning the most amazing fundraiser this weekend. Would love to have you there! ☺ Please Share! ☺"

The post has received 73 Likes and 5 Shares in the time it takes me to pass one level of Candy Crush and for the first time today, I notice that I have again made a dramatic leap in Likers, passing the 4,000-mark and getting mostly positive comments on my wall.

Diana thinks she's found the perfect venue for the exhibition, and Hell Pa has sent me a photo of the first completed painting in the *Nude Male Cleaners of the World* series, and all of this is a nice distraction from the meeting that's looming over me, shadowing me like a giant's steel-capped boot, absorbing all my attention, but it's simply not enough and that's why I find myself getting out of the car and walking towards Paul.

'Hello, Joel,' he says, lifting his hand, without turning his head to look at me.

'Hello, Paul,' I say, standing next to him, lifting my hand and staring across the children's crossing to the other side of the road.

'It's a beautiful day,' he says, in a monotone way. He seems…not nervous but…*stilted*. As if he's *practicing* having a conversation.

'It's a beautiful day,' I say, repeating him, not really certain of how to continue.

'Yes,' he says, rising up on the balls of his feet a little and then planting his feet again. 'Cocksucker.'

Across the road, pressed into the gutter by some hardened mud and leaves, is a blue ribbon flapping in the breeze that a pupil has obviously lost after receiving first place for something in school sports. I have this desire to go and pluck it free, but I simply can't while Paul is watching. I'm yawning and rising on to the balls of my feet and the whimpering of Barnaby is suddenly so annoying to me that I imagine rolling crushed glass into mincemeat or maybe just deleting the Virtual Dog app from my phone – even though I'd never do either of those things in reality – and it's just as I've finished toileting Barnaby, so that he's wagging his tail with his tongue hanging out, that Sylvia finally arrives.

'See you, Paul,' I say.

'See you, Joel,' he says.

Sylvia and I meet at the school gate and I almost fall into her; I'm so happy to see her. So much seems to have happened since this morning.

'I feel like I haven't seen you for ages,' I say, hugging her, my face in her hair.

'Me, too. Look,' she says, holding her phone towards me so I can see the dick pic – thighs, abs, shoulder, everything except for the male face – that I sent her after I left Jen's this morning.

'Oh. Oops. That's not what I wanted to show you,' she says, looking at her phone, swiping, tapping, then pausing to just stare at me. 'I loved that photo by the way. And how you described it was just…wow…I mean…how is it that you can't write a blog post to save yourself, but you can write such short descriptive amazing things about the pictures you're sending me? You really turn me on.'

'Maybe I just don't panic as much when you're with me…or when I'm thinking of you.'

'Anyway,' she says, as we walk inside the school gates and start the countdown to the meeting. 'What I meant to show you was *this*.'

She opens a text without actually holding the phone up to me this time, but I can see by the display that it's from a number that is not stored in her contacts. "'Hey there Sylvia,'" she reads "'had such a great time last night. You guys rock. I was wondering if it might be okay if I moved in today? I have my bags packed. Can be over there soon. Doug.'"

'Oh my God,' I say, another pang of nerves, but a different kind. 'When did he send that?'

'This morning,' she says. 'I was too busy to think about it or text you. What do you think?'

'We have an insanely big house. It's almost impossible to say no,' I say, almost choking, hitting myself in the chest. 'Text "yes" and choose the party hat emoji. I mean…no. *Wait!* It's too much. Just use the *smiley face* emoticon. No. In fact, don't use any emoji or an emoticon at all. Just text "yes".'

We reach the classroom and peep through the windows and I notice Dylan first of all and am surprised to see him actually joining in with all the other kids who are packing up equipment around little tables, where they were obviously using Clag to make pictures out of what looks like glitter and streamers and icy-pole sticks.

I try to calm down, to disassociate myself from my awkwardness, to find that sense of goadiness that carried me through the confrontation at the gym, but when I say, 'Wow, multi-coloured icy pole sticks,' Sylvia can see through me right away and whispers, 'Don't worry. Just watch me and see how I handle this. I deal with conflict head-on every day at work. It's what I'm employed for.'

'They're trying to change him,' I say, pointing as he runs to the mat and crosses his legs like all the other kids. 'Look at him. He doesn't do that. It's like he's been *drugged*. They can't just…shame someone into line like that.'

Sylvia says, 'Listen. Just follow my lead, okay? You'll calm down if you just let me take the lead,' but she is unable to turn my face towards hers because I'm transfixed, suspended in disbelief, as I watch the children gathering in front of the woman who's sitting on a chair with a book in her hand.

'*Multi-Mum*'s in there,' I whisper.

'What?' Sylvia says, leaning in closer to the window. 'The one that called you a pervert? That bitch is *Multi-Mum*? What the fuck's she doing here?'

'They knew we were coming today. Mrs. Brogan must realise that this is…that this is…this feels like…this feels like a *set-up*. Jesus Christ,' I say, freaked out, flipping the cover on my iPhone. 'I have to feed Barnaby.'

Sylvia flips the cover back over and holds my hand tight.

'Stay cool and calm,' she says, revealing something new to me in the way her eyes peel open as she focuses in on *Multi-Mum*, the way she sneers and then thins her lips out; the way she seems to reel back on her haunches like a big orange tom cat who's run into another big orange tom cat down some cobble-stoned alley between two houses, and it suddenly occurs to me that I've never seen her performing in her work environment, that I don't really ever see her under those kinds of stressful conditions.

She's never been to the school for a meeting before, in fact has never even *met* Mrs. Brogan. But she *has* met many very powerful business people on the very top floors of high-rise buildings in cities all over the world to negotiate deals where *millions* of dollars are on the line, and what was I worrying about, *seriously?* This is a meeting in a small suburban school with a replaceable school principal, a likable teacher of five- and six-year-old children, and a thirty-dollar-an-hour psychologist, and there is not *one* person in that preppy little threesome who Sylvia can't eat for *breakfast*.

'Just watch me and you'll be okay,' she says again, in a manner that's so familiar. I'm spinning in *déjà vu*, trying to place the last time I heard her speak this way to me. It's distracting enough that whatever was blocking my ability to proceed is suddenly released or removed. A deep breath opens me up and calms me down and I'm projecting forward to the end of the meeting, imagining Sylvia and I smirk-glaring at *Multi-Mum*, walking away from the school after shaking hands in a contained victorious way, having advocated for Dylan at the same time that we robbed them of all their stinky smugness.

We open the door and walk in and when we turn the corner into the classroom, the heads of all the kids swivel towards us. Dylan smiles and I smile back, but the silvery paper of two dozen Clag-bound jellyfish hanging from the ceiling reflect sunlight into my eyes, forcing me to duck my head a little and turn left. There's Mrs. Brogan, sitting at a small round table which is partially obscured by two rows of metal book shelves filled with file boxes of thin books.

I wave, stupidly, when she motions me over to the two empty chairs before holding my hand out towards Sylvia. I'm surprised to see her squatting beside Dylan on the reading mat, kissing his head and hugging him, and I'm still waiting with my hand out towards her when she stands up to stare at *Multi-Mum* with such a fierce indifference that *Multi-Mum* lowers her gaze, opens the book – *Spot Goes to the Farm* – and pretends to be having trouble finding the first page.

There are white patches in my vision as we walk behind the metal cabinets and discover that Mrs. Fox and the psychologist are also at the table. I'm happy to be able to lean back and see Dylan from where I'm sitting, and I notice he's glancing my way, smiling, and I remember our agreement about the iPhone, relieved to know that he's only *pretending* to be like the other kids.

The psychologist is smiling, condescendingly, of course, as she pulls a thick report of some kind from a manila folder and after noticing that there are only four phones on the table, I'm bewildered that she doesn't seem to have one. As we shuffle through two minutes of small talk – we're being buttered up – I notice Sylvia's hands are shaking and get *déjà vu* again.

She clasps her hands together on the table in front of her and glares at Mrs. Brogan who seems so large – the biggest of all of us – as she explains that Dylan was so disruptive last week, he had to spend an hour in her office. With her chin lifted, she claims some insight into our life, into my very psyche, by telling us, 'When I got down on my knees and looked him in the eyes, he calmed down immediately and this approach has *always* worked with my *daughter*. Sometimes, children just need consistency from their parents if they're going to settle down and fit in.'

She has her head tilted as she's saying this, a know-it-all smile on her face, and all of a sudden, I'm burning from the inside out, imaging all these horrific things I'll never actually do to her in reality, trying to come up with a way to respond to her comment because it offends me *deeply* somehow, distracted the whole time by the way *Multi-Mum* is reading to the children.

Why the fuck is she rounding her words like she isn't a fucking bogan like the rest of us? Why is she reading to my son like she *hasn't* started a social media campaign to defame me, like she *hasn't* called me a pervert, like she isn't using my honest Internet posting error to turn me into a villain she can build her faux-outrage against, getting more Shares and more Likes by playing the self-righteous social media warrior, the community-minded *super* parent, championing same sex marriage when she knows – she'd know for *certain* – that I aligned myself to that particular social issue last *January*, way before it was even really popular?

And it's as I'm becoming more and more astounded at her tactical nous – she's obviously attempting to distance my gay followers from me so that she can steal them for herself – that I become more specifically aware of why I'm burning so deeply after Mrs. Brogan's comment.

'Our son is not *your* daughter,' I say, which doesn't explain what I mean at all, and after another attempt, saying, 'I've been with Dylan every day for six years…' and then stopping and trying once again, 'Not everyone needs to *fit in*,' but not even getting *close* to what I'm *feeling* inside, I just give in, attempt to coach myself through this nightmare meeting while also attempting to harness myself around Gus's words – *You have to become more aware of people around you* – but actually feeling that I'm *too* aware of other people around me. The urge to reach for my phone, which is vibrating and offering me something restorative, is almost too strong to ignore.

"*Calm down, Joel,*" I say to myself, as my phone falls silent. "*Just calm down and watch Sylvia. Just watch Sylvia.*"

It becomes obvious that, while I've been scrambling inside to recover myself, Sylvia has been talking with the psychologist, who's flipping over to the last page on the report, pointing to certain columns and rows, circling certain paragraphs with her finger.

When I hear *Multi-Mum*'s voice shorten in anger, I lean back to see a young girl, Rebecca, I think, over at a box of Legos, pulling pieces out and crying for some reason. Two boys are wrestling on the edge of the group, banging into the trundle wheels of the whiteboard, and Dylan is just sitting there.

When I try to focus back on the report, the psychologist is suddenly speaking in a very apologetic way as she taps on a particular number in the very last row in the very last column, and I realise I missed something here because everyone sitting at the round table seems tense.

The *déjà vu* comes again when I see blotches of red appearing on Sylvia's neck and on her cheeks and the Mrs. Brogan-fuelled *rage* I was feeling only moments ago is suddenly expressed perfectly in the skin pinching over the bridge of Sylvia's nose, the redemptive sheen in her eyes, the sliver of clenched teeth I can see through the left side of her mouth, her lips thin straight clean lines, barely open.

It's not until I see her fingers unthreading, her hands fluttering visibly through the air to find stillness; one landing over the psychological report, one clasping the edge of the table in front of me, that I notice the white-shock in her knuckles and remember why Sylvia's pre-meeting attempt to calm me felt so familiar. I remember us boarding the plane together again, heading for one of her first business conferences in Barcelona.

I'd never flown before and was sweating, bumbling, certain we were going to die.

'Just watch me,' she'd said. 'I fly all the time. Just watch me if you feel scared and you'll see that there's nothing to worry about and you'll calm down,' and for the first four hours of the twenty-two-hour flight, I just watched her, and watched her until – soothed by her constant smile and the smooth flight – I almost forgot we were in the air and started chatting with her, ordering drinks, watching movies, so amazed at how terrified and childish I'd been for the days leading up to the flight that I even laughed at myself.

But then, we began our descent, dipping below the clouds into a violent storm where we experienced such terrifying turbulence that the plane dropped and rose with enough force to make our feet leave the floor. My belt bruised me and everyone, including the flight attendants, screamed.

As we approached the runway, we swung heavily to the left and then heavily to the right and at the point where I needed the most encouragement, when I desperately needed some visual confirmation that we were going to be okay, the plane slammed into the runway, giving me whiplash, and then rebounded and landed, and rebounded and landed, again and again.

Through my terror, as I was screaming in a pitch I had no idea I was capable of, I turned to Sylvia for that sense of calm, to see her gripping the seat in front of her, eyes closed so tight her eyeballs seemed to have been scooped out, her entire face wet from tears and streaked black with makeup, her mouth open as wide as I've even seen it before or since, her tongue actually pushing out as if she was dehydrated and just hoping for a miraculous drop of water to appear out of nowhere, so totally hysterical that her nose started suddenly bleeding, streaming around her lips and dripping from her chin, her prolonged screeching breaking on impact and reforming as we rebounded from the tarmac another several times. And I was certain, as I've ever been, that we were going to die.

The psychological report is partially torn and thrown into the air, and the psychologist baulks heavily in her chair as Sylvia propels herself forward, leaning into the table so that two of the four legs lift of the floor and cause the table to wail out a loud cracking sound and the first thing I think, as I stand and put an arm out in front of Sylvia – by nothing more than reflex, really – is that the psychologist looks way too shocked and frightened for someone who's supposed to be *practiced* in the extremes of human emotion.

I'm forced to stand up because Mrs. Brogan has risen from her chair with her arms above her head like a riled freaking bear, saying, 'Sylvia, *please*,' in such a strange way – like a whispering chainsaw – and so I also raise *my* arms in the air, surprised that I not only match her reach, but *surpass* it, most likely because of the superior flexibility in my shoulder girdles.

Mrs. Fox is just sitting there with her eyebrows raised, completely still, like the wax museum version of herself, and as the psychologist screams, 'Call the doctor!' Sylvia spins to face Mrs. Brogan and attempts to rush her but is so mindless now that she's forgotten about the table between them and, after banging her thighs into it, is thrust backward into the chair so that it tips over. She crashes to the floor on her back, accidentally performing an impressive reverse somersault and flinging one of her shoes into the kinetic sand boxes over by the school bags.

'I mean, call the *police*,' the psychologist screams, her hands balled into tiny little fists in front of her, exposing a tear in the sleeve of her cardigan, which I assume Sylvia's responsible for.

Sylvia stumbles back to her feet, her blouse half unbuttoned, raging, and my intention is to simply calm her down, but she grabs hold of my upper arm as I reach for her and uses my weight as an anchor, propelling herself into the air, landing in the middle of the table on her knees, legs spread wide for balance, snatching at Mrs. Brogan's necklace in what I can only assume is a mindless, *unplanned* move.

'Joel's a good father!' she says, chainsaw-whispering just as Mrs. Brogan did and…I'm just suddenly so *grateful*. Sylvia is as offended by the inference of bad parenting as I am.

But Sylvia's different to me. While I sit idly by fuming inside, fumbling for words, merely *imagining* the horrible things I might do to Mrs. Brogan – and to that nattering, wafer-brained, cardigan-wearing psychologist who's using some arbitrary test to project a deficit or delay on to our perfectly gorgeous son – Sylvia's getting out of her chair and actually *doing* those horrible things.

It appears that Sylvia gets blood noses whenever she's hyped to a certain level of mania because she's bleeding again, just like she was on the plane, and I think it's this that causes Mrs. Brogan to make a gargling sound, to take hold of Sylvia's wrist with both hands, to start swinging her shoulders violently in an attempt to free herself.

The table cracks so loudly that Mrs. Fox says 'Wow,' looking straight ahead without any facial expression whatsoever, and the psychologist is pressed up against the metal book shelves, her balled fists and torn cardigan in front of her bowed head screaming 'Call, call, call' and I have my cheek against Sylvia's back, hugging her, loving her, attempting to pull her free from Mrs. Brogan's vise-like grip, *feeling* more than thinking, that this is the difference between women like Sylvia, who shake down international business meetings and make a demonstrable difference to world economies, and men like *me*, who benefit the world in a less practical way that's not even really measurable. Ours is almost the perfect pairing. There's a kind of destiny revealing itself here – how Sylvia's pulling me into this real world moment; how I'm holding her back to prevent her from going too far.

The table is collapsing. I'm stepping away with the full weight of Sylvia in my arms and although I'm not bigger than Mrs. Brogan *physically*, I am somehow bigger in *every other way* as long as Sylvia's here.

'We'll home school him! Is that what you want?' I say, and that chainsaw whisper makes sense to me now, because we're all trying to keep this confrontation from the children. I look over my shoulder and there's *Multi-Mum* huddling them in the corner near the whiteboard, holding her phone in our direction.

'You want us to fucking home-school him?' I whisper-scream again, and suddenly, the air is warmer. It's as if Sylvia and I are on top of a mountain, hand in hand, watching a volcano erupting in the distance. We're going to perish and be fossilised in a bed of cooling lava. The two of us together.

Sylvia, who has somehow taken off her other shoe, holding the high heel in front of her like it's a hunting knife, manages to calm down enough that I allow her feet to touch the ground.

Mrs. Fox says 'Well, this was a first,' as Sylvia collects her other shoe and puts both of them on, with a surprisingly nonchalant kind of smile.

The psychologist stops screaming 'call' and Mrs. Brogan just stops, seems to hold her breath. Everything slows and becomes muffled to the sound of a single prolonged heartbeat.

I'm right beside Sylvia as we pick up our phones from the floor. After tearing away some absorbent towelling from one of the craft buckets and pushing it into her hand, I tell her to wait outside, that I'll collect Dylan.

When I turn to the children and hold out my hand, I'm blinded by the glittery jellyfish again so that Dylan just appears from the glaze, smiling, to take hold of two of my fingers.

He leads me to the school bags and after he's collected his bag and some really poorly done artwork, I look back one more time to see *Multi-Mum* still holding her phone in our direction. Getting my goadiness back, I lift *my* phone and point it in *her* direction and after staying like that for a moment or two, say, 'I've scheduled Hell Pa's art exhibition to clash with your sausage sizzle. There'll be a lot of nude art…a lot of gay people there. We're going to make a lot of money. A lot more money than *you*. And we're going to donate it all to the school.'

'You're insane,' *Multi-Mum* says. 'You're just totally insane.'

'I'm insanely happy,' I say. 'Sausage Sizzler.'

There are dark clouds over us suddenly, and two mothers already waiting outside the classroom for the final school bell and I'm surprised to see them talking to Sylvia, who's standing there with her nose covered in the blood-clogged absorbent towelling, nodding, rolling her eyes, receiving what looks like sympathy – one of the mothers has her hand on Sylvia's shoulder – and after Dylan runs to her and says, 'Mummy, what happened to your nose?' she rolls her eyes again and says, 'Mummy just got a little silly, Dyl' before catching my gaze and mouthing, 'Oops.'

She thanks the two mums, and I nod at them as she waves goodbye and I can hear them whispering excitedly as we cross the quadrangle.

Sylvia says 'I think I totally—'

'*Lost* it?' I say, looking up at the sky, feeling drops of rain on my face. 'Yep.'

'Yeah,' she says, with a laugh that sounds like a hiccup. 'I think I basically assaulted Principal…whatever her name was.'

'I only saw you holding her necklace,' I say, as we reach the end of the grassy area between the playground and the sandpit and there's Paul in the middle of the road.

He holds his hand up and says, 'Hello, Joel', as if I hadn't just seen him twenty minutes ago. I notice something poking out of the top of the hand that's gripping the stop sign, as the rain begins to really tumble down, and I feel compelled to run and meet him as he reaches the curb.

'Why are you holding that?' I say, eyeing the end of the blue ribbon I'd seen in the gutter.

'Hello, Joel,' he says, handing it to me, so that goose bumps charge over my back and neck in a way that can only be described as pleasant, emotional.

We are under the gaze of others as we walk the footpath, and every set of eyes we pass focusses on Sylvia's bloody nose, and then on me, before turning quickly away. When we reach the cars, Sylvia says, 'I hope I haven't stuffed things up,' and seems on the verge of tears.

I shake my head, stop her, turn her towards me, thanking her in the way I do up the buttons on her shirt, thanking her by the way I look into her eyes and pull her hair into the shape of a pony tail, smoothing all the strands together.

After I kiss her on the forehead and pull her in for a hug, Dylan runs into our legs *hard*, wraps his arms around us, buries his head in.

The Cloud

85:39:21

It takes more time than I thought it would to buckle Dylan into his seat, to check two notifications on my phone – the first from Twitter: **"@Aaannne** just retweeted @dadinating's Tweet"; the second from Facebook: *"D-D-Dad's* post 'Some people are so insecure…' is performing better than 95% of other posts on that Page" – and to open the Virtual Dog app so that Dylan can feed Barnaby on the way home.

By the time we've pulled away from the curb, six minutes have passed and Sylvia is long gone and I have to resist the urge to take my phone back from Dylan so that I can text her a smiley face emoticon.

'Dad,' Dylan says. 'Brandon can't pretend.'

'He can't?'

'Mrs. Fox put him in the corner and he cried.'

'Oh,' I say. 'Poor Brandon.'

'Rebecca can't pretend, as well.'

'Was that Rebecca pulling out all the Legos?' I ask, as I hit several pre-set buttons on the radio and stop on Taylor Swift's song 'Wildest Dreams'. It's mid-way though and I let it linger for a while, surprised to find that it resonates with me on some level. It's kind of…*happy-sad.*

'*I can* pretend,' Dylan says, head down, concentrating.

'You were sitting very still. You had your legs crossed. You were listening,' I say. 'You must *really* want that iPhone.'

'Can I have it now?'

We turn left and then left again and I really am in a hurry to get back home to see how Sylvia's feeling and so reach instinctively to the passenger seat, the console, and then between my legs before remembering that Dylan has my phone. When I hear it quack, I find it kind of cute, like it knew I was looking for it.

'Mummy texted,' Dylan says, as I turn on the windscreen wipers and look up into the clouds, which are so low and dark to the point of being almost black.

'Hey, Dylan. There's a big storm coming. You can see lightening already. Look!'

'No,' he says.

'Sebastian's mum is bad,' I say, so rapidly that I surprise myself. 'What do you think of Sebastian?'

'I don't like Sebastian,' he says, monotone, and by the sound of Barnaby's barking, the way he's panting, I can tell that Dylan's using one of the dozen dog toys I've earned or bought, and it's a relief that someone else is looking after him for a change, really giving him attention, because the last time I took him to the virtual vet, he'd lost one kilogram and his coat had dropped from 100% to 92% sheen. I lost thirty thousand points and couldn't afford to buy him the most expensive kennel, as I'd planned.

'You don't have to like everyone, Dylan. You just have to be *liked*…by everyone,' I say, trailing into a whisper, only mouthing the last two words, wondering where this actually came from, wondering if I actually believe it.

'I like Audrey. And I like Mrs. Fox.'

'You like Mrs. Fox?' I say, surprised.

'Yes,' he says.

The wipers are swishing across the windscreen on their highest setting as I reach over to the passenger seat, as my desire to get home to Sylvia makes me push the pointer on the speedometer above fifty. 'Well, you don't have to worry about school now, Dyl. You don't have to pretend anymore. I'm going to home school you now.'

'What's home school?'

'It means I'm going to teach you about everything,' I say, turning the headlights on when I notice cars coming from the opposite direction have turned on theirs. 'And that you're not going to go to school anymore.'

Another quick glance into the rear vision mirror as I'm turning the corner into our street and I catch Dylan staring at me in a way that makes me hold my breath and I know by the way he places the phone down next to him and stares out the window – even before he says 'I don't want to home school' – that I've made an error, but there's no time to talk about it right now because we're pulling into the driveway as Taylor Swift is singing and there's Sylvia in the garage standing next to the car talking to Doug, who has two bags hanging over his shoulder and a large suitcase beside him.

Dylan takes off through the garage and into the house without even stopping to say hello, and I'm worried because I don't know if he's upset. I'm already imagining myself apologising to Mrs. Brogan somehow, so that he can continue going to school, but all that gets pushed aside as I approach Sylvia and Doug. I know that Sylvia will be feeling, well, just a little self-conscious talking to Doug with her face and work shirt covered in blood.

There is clear awkwardness in the way I reach out to shake Doug's hand, and I'm sure he picks up on it even though he's smiling broadly as he says hello, chuckling while commenting on the events at Dylan's school. I'm not sure if Sylvia has told him part of the story, or the full story, or even made something up and so I say nothing, not even hello.

When he accepts my handshake – skin on skin – I try not to think of the haunted house, the way Sylvia manipulated me there, the size of Doug's cock and how close I was to having it in my mouth, and then, for some reason, I'm drawn to the way Doug is dressed, which he obviously picks up on because he touches the black bowtie and runs his hand down his white shirt and says, 'I had an audition in the city.'

'I'm going to have a shower,' Sylvia says, smiling, but because she appears more than just a *little* self-conscious, I text "I'll be upstairs ASAP" after she walks through the garage door into the house, and after putting my iPhone in my pocket, slinging Dylan's school bag over my shoulder, I pick up Doug's suitcase and guide him into the house.

'We'll put your bags in the hallway and I'll show you around and after you've chosen a room—'

'Is Sylvia okay?' Doug says, following me into the hall where I hear Dylan talking with someone who I mistake for Monica at first, before realising the voice is slightly deeper. 'If this isn't a good time, I can just head back to Sean's house.'

I don't really know Doug, but I'm struck by how much I want him to be here, and after dismissing his concern in a good-natured way, I tell him he'll have to get used to a little bit of craziness if he's going to survive even one night with us and it's at that point, where Doug laughs and I feel the awkwardness abating a little, that I walk him in to Hell Pa's art studio with the intention of introducing him to Dylan, Dad, and Monica, only to find that the room has changed.

The mattress has been pushed under the bedroom window and there are black sheets strung up on one wall, black confetti covering the carpet, and black streamers hanging from the roof and, standing dead centre in all of this blackness, is a naked woman with long blonde hair, a slender face, bright, round green eyes – which I feel immediately attracted to – and large boobs that have obviously been surgically enhanced. She's holding a large white stuffed toy which, at first glance, I think is a baby seal before noticing the carrot and the top hat and realising it's a *snowman*.

I make eye contact with Dad, who's standing by the easel with Dylan, when Doug stops behind me and says, 'Okay,' in a way that sounds more like a question than an affirmation.

'Dad paints nudes,' I say, rolling my eyes, before I notice that Doug is smiling, bemused, his eyes levelled at the woman's crotch, and I don't know if it was the slightly odd-shaped boobs that distracted me from this, but the female love model Dad is painting right at this moment has a cock and balls.

After staring into the live model's eyes, looking at the live models cock and balls, looking at Dylan, and then back into the live model's eyes, I say, 'Dad?'

'This is Taylor.'

'Taylor?' I say. 'Like Taylor Swift?'

'I was a Taylor way before Taylor Swift,' Taylor says, shaking her head, dropping her arms to her side, holding the snowman in one hand, her cock swinging a little bit. 'But I like her music.'

'I was hoping Taylor could move in with us for a while,' Dad says, turning away from the canvas to face me. 'I'm going to paint her for the exhibition. I have a lot of ideas.'

'Oh, you're asking for our permission this time?' I say, a little snarky as my phone quacks a text message, which I assume will be from Sylvia, but is actually from Jen. "Are you guys okay?" it says. "I heard you got in a fight with Mrs. Brogan" and I'm distracted enough to start texting her back while saying, 'Where did you find a shemale?'

'Not *shemale*,' Dad says, so that I stop texting and look up to see him mouthing *sorry* to Taylor. He seems so embarrassed and disappointed in me that I flip the cover of my phone closed.

'I don't like that term,' Taylor says, hands still by her side.

'Taylor's transgender,' Doug says.

'Taylor's transgender,' I say.

'Shemale's *derogatory*,' she says. 'And anyway, I'm just Taylor.'

'It's often *shemale* on the Internet,' I say, so that Doug laughs and Taylor just stands there and despite having just met, she looks as disappointed in me as Dad does. 'Did you and Dad…*connect* on Craigslist?'

'You left Sylvia's account open again,' Dad says. 'And I just thought a transgender model would be perfect.

There's the ambiguity of gender and…what were you saying, Taylor?'

'We need to see more art and more stories about people who don't identify as cis,' she says.

'Cis? I say. 'What's a cis?'

'Cisgender is like you,' Taylor says. 'You were born male and identify as male. I was born a male but identify as female. There's more to gender than just genitals.'

'And it's really popular on Facebook now,' Dad says. 'I'm surprised you haven't heard of it.'

'I promote gay rights,' I say to Taylor, feeling frustrated, annoyed, distracted, thinking of Sylvia. 'And also marriage *equality*.'

'Well, why not promote the rights of everyone?' she says, hands up, hands down, leaning forward. Face, boobs, cock.

Taylor's expression softens just a little – possibly because she can see my utter confusion – and she stands upright, holding the snowman in front of her so that its big white head covers her genitals and she's suddenly a woman. She's suddenly a woman *only*.

'And just in terms of becoming a more skilful painter,' Dad says, shaking me from a moment of reverie, awakening my frustration. 'With Taylor here, I can get a visual on every body part.'

'Oh, you can get a visual on *every* body part, can you?' I say. 'You've got breasts and you've got a penis. Anything missing? You think? How about the vagina, Dad? Where's the vagina?'

'Here I am,' Monica says, her hand appearing from between the mattress and the doona. 'Sleeping.'

Doug's laughing as Dylan walks over and pulls the doona back to expose Monica's head, and when she blinks into the light and says, 'Hello, sweetheart Dylan,' I feel strangely moved. I feel like I'm in a rocket that's taking off, hovering, taking off again, hovering, taking off again.

'Are you the new cleaner?' Dad asks, looking curiously at Doug, crossing his arms and eyeing him up and down, the paintbrush pointing towards the ceiling.

'Oh…no,' I say, realising that Dad was making assumptions based on Doug's clothing. 'He was at an audition.'

'I was a dancing waiter,' Doug says. 'I'm Doug.'

Monica squeals, sits up, and after partially wrapping herself in the doona, runs over, throws one arm around Doug's neck, and tiptoes up to hug him. 'It's so amazing to meet you.'

'Hello, Doug,' Dad says, shaking his hand warmly, and then hugging him, actually *hugging* him, as if he's meeting a great friend of mine who I've been talking about with affection for many years and *not* a guy we found on Craigslist who I rode a sea-themed carousel with less than twenty-four hours ago. The awkwardness comes rushing back when he says, 'We're so grateful for what you're doing for Joel.'

Doug looks from Dad to me and he appears to be, well, *loving* this, and I remember the way Jen behaved when she first came into our home, as if she was walking around in a brand new world, in awe.

'And I thought living with a bunch of *exotic dancers* would be the strangest experience of my life,' Doug says.

'You're moving in with us?' Monica asks, picking up Dylan and spinning around with him, cheering when he answers yes.

Taylor picks up a robe and slips into it slowly, and my eyes shift from her face to her boobs to her cock before she's covered up fully. The fact that I am attracted to her, that my eyes have followed that path down her body several times since we entered the room, comes almost as an afterthought.

'Hell Pa,' Doug says, in a way that commands all our attention as he leans one canvas – a painting of a staircase that spirals upwards towards a bright moon with a breast on every step – away from the wall, to retrieve the painting behind it. 'Are these your paintings? They're great.'

'I'm getting much better.' Dad stands behind Doug with his hands on his hips to admire his own painting, which is an extreme close-up of a vagina that takes up the entire canvas. A little man is running into the vulva – presented as a long black tunnel – while looking over his shoulder, as if being chased by something. 'Monica modelled for this one.'

I focus away from the expression on the man's face which is poorly painted, as are most of Dad's paintings, after deciding that he was trying to depict either terror or pleasure, or maybe serenity, or perhaps *revulsion*, to text Jen that Sylvia and I are okay, that it wasn't such a big deal at the school anyway, and in the time it takes Hell Pa to say, 'That's me. You can't tell?' in response to whatever Doug said, I receive her reply which reads, "There were police at the school".

'Yeah, of course,' Doug says. 'I knew it was you. I love this one.'

'Me, too,' Hell Pa says. 'This is definitely going in the exhibition.'

This yawn may be the result of tiredness, *exhaustion*, or this yawn may be the result of nervous energy, *fear* but every crazy turn in my mind is suddenly leading me to Sylvia, and as Doug asks about the exhibition, I say, 'Monica, can you show Doug around for me? Help him to pick a room? And introduce him to Diana. And Dylan, you stay with Hell Pa. I'm just going to go see Mummy.'

'Diana's on her way back,' Hell Pa says. 'She's found an amazing venue. And it's available for this Sunday. I've posted a pic on the Hell Pa Facebook page.'

'Great,' I say, texting "fuck" back to Jen, then wishing I hadn't.

'Are you okay, Joel?' Dad says, so that everyone focuses in on me, in silence.

'Who's ever really okay?' I say, a forced chuckle to make it seem like it's not a serious question.

This sadness comes with a smile and an awareness of all of us together. Hell Pa running terrified into vulvas, Monica modelling for food and a place to stay, Dylan pretending for an iPhone, Taylor cornered by gender, Doug unable to forgive his mother, and me, unable to forgive my father. We're all on the ground like this, all on the Internet like that, and all in the universe – the 'cloud' now – like everything.

'Welcome, Doug and Taylor. Welcome *home*,' I say, opening my Instagram app and saying 'smile', so that everyone bunches in together, staring through the black streamers, Doug still holding the painting, Taylor with her hand on Dylan's head.

I share this picture to all of my social media accounts, tagging in several Facebook pages, referencing Dad's painting and flagging the exhibition, before I finish climbing the steps towards Sylvia.

HE SHOULD OPEN UP A SHOP

86:21:53

Sylvia's sitting against the bedhead wearing shorts and a T-shirt with her hair damp and uncombed, the back of her hand against her knee, tapping into her phone which rings as I sit down beside her.

She puts it to her ear, mouths *sorry* while waving at me with her fingers, and then puts her free hand on my thigh, saying, 'Hey,' to whoever's called her. 'Yeah…it was crazy. Remember when we ran into those girls after the Christmas party? Kind of like that only with more…*venom.*'

I assume Sylvia's talking to one of her work colleagues. There's laughter as I hold my phone out, displaying Jen's text, so that Silvia sits up to read it. 'Oh, the police went to the school, apparently'.

There's more laughter, and I'm surprised to see Sylvia laughing, as well, in a way that seems a little hysterical, like a school girl who's sat up too late with her friends eating chocolate and popcorn and drinking Red Bull, and so I send her a text which reads, "I thought you'd be upset about the police".

Sylvia says, 'Hang on, Jacqui. I got a text,' checks her phone, then looks at me and shrugs as if the presence of police and the whole scene at school was no big deal at all and so I text, "Multi-Mum was filming the whole thing on her phone. She'll probably YouTube it".

While Sylvia apologises to Jacqui again and takes her phone from her ear to read it, I open my Facebook app, hold my breath as I search for *Multi-Mum*, only breathing out when I see that there's no recently posted video there.

'Oh my God. *Multi-Mum* videoed it. It's probably going to be on YouTube,' Sylvia says.

Jacqui screams *yes* through the phone, and there's more hysterical laughter, and when I open my Pages app, I see that my Likers have increased *again*, to 4,171. I'm pretty chuffed about that until I notice that I've been tagged into a post by Hell Pa because it's revealed to me that my pens-and-paper, old world father has more Likers than me, a staggering 16,444. All sense of importance, all sense of *achievement*, all the years of effort I put into presenting myself in a certain way in order to build a following of people who liked that sort of person, is wiped away like suds off a recently washed window.

I stand up and start pacing a horseshoe shape around the bed, scrolling through some of Hell Pa's old posts, more depressed than angry as I see the engagement he's been getting – so many Likes, so many comments, so many Shares – and I'm dipping in and out of Sylvia's conversation, missing most of it, in despair at Dad amassing such a huge following in such a small amount of time. It's only when I go back to the start of his feed to see if one of his posts was shared by George Takei or something, that I see the picture he tagged me in. It's the venue Diana found for the exhibition, which looks very cool – a long, narrow building with plenty of wall space for hanging paintings and a wooden stage at the very end. 224 Cooper Street, only half a block away from *Multi-Mum*'s sausage sizzle.

'If it wasn't for Joel, I might have strangled her to death or something,' Silvia says, giggling, reaching out with her foot in an attempt to get my attention as I pace the floor, tapping my phone. 'Oh, well, Dylan's probably not so suited to school, anyway. So Joel's going to home school him.'

After copying and pasting the address of the venue, I open the Facebook event I created, titled *The Hell Pa Art Exhibition Fundraiser for Limesgrown East Primary School*, make some small changes to the event description, and with a burst of certainty that convinces me it's okay to post it without running it by Sylvia first, the event is live. It's on. We're doing this.

Hey all my friends and family and great fans,

My dad, Hell Pa, is not the greatest artist. But he's trying hard and already has more than 16,000 followers on Facebook so that tells me he's genuine. For the first time in his life he's genuine. He must have something going for him. Since discovering the Internet he has found love, painted nudes, including male cleaners, a transgender named Taylor and a recently acquired girlfriend named Monica, and he is happier now (he tried to kill himself as a retired banker). He's an example of how anyone can change, even 70-year-olds. Without further ado, I want to announce the exhibition we're running this Saturday, which will display all Hell Pa's paintings for sale. All money raised will go to the Limesgrown East Primary School to paint the bike sheds and improve the cracks in the asphalt. ☺ !!Please Like and Share!! ☺

I'm still pacing around the bed as I post it, but as I tag in about a dozen pages who follow me including *Gay Cops*, *Bisexual Community Apps*, *Wickedly Hot Men*, and *Playgroups Australia*, I hear Sylvia tell Jacqui, 'Yeah, he's amazing,' and I find myself slowing down, lifting my gaze from the phone, becoming less reactive.

'Send it through to me,' Sylvia says. 'That sounds like the perfect job for him.'

A Twitter notification tells me that "@feedingjen and @DrChrisGibbons just retweeted a photo" and I'm opening it, conscious I haven't Tweeted much in the past few days, hoping it will be something *I* can also retweet, when I hear Sylvia clicking her fingers in the air, still talking on the phone, her legs spreading open in a relaxed but purposeful manner. With her hand still in the air, she points towards her pussy and nods at me, her cheeks suddenly flushed.

'Really?' I mouth, conscious that she's still talking to Jacqui, cock swelling.

'No, send me through the whole article,' she says into the phone, pulling the soft cotton material of her shorts aside so that her pussy is right there, no underwear.

I can hear the murmuring of Monica touring Doug around the house as I lie down and slip my phoneless hand through the leg hole of her shorts, reaching past the elastic waist band to touch her belly button before dragging my fingers down over the sexy hairy mound, as slowly as possible, my thumb and little finger gliding down opposite thighs, two fingers running over her lips, my middle finger over her clit and slit. 'He's so great with his hands,' she says, her breathing deeper, but her voice the same. 'He'll build up a regular clientele in no time.'

It's disappointing that she's had a shower because her natural scent is gone and this may be the reason I'm not losing my mind like I usually do, but it doesn't really matter because everything else is there – the way her thighs make me feel safely enclosed, the soft, hot wet of her pussy, the way it feels to be beneath her like this, the potential to become narrowed down to the point of being almost thoughtless.

I'm fuelled by wonder and curiosity as she says, 'I can guarantee an orgasm for every woman who walks through the door' and when I wrap my other arm around her thigh, my phone still in my hand, I ignore the Facebook notification – hoping it's one of the tagged pages sharing my event – and move my hand over her, slowly, several times in a row, covering as much skin as possible, from her belly to her pussy and as close to her asshole as possible.

Each time my hand returns to her belly, my middle finger comes up wetter than before, so I hold my middle finger at her opening licking very lightly around the lips of her pussy, over her clit, pausing to brush my teeth against her inner thighs, closing my mouth into a kiss as I slide my finger into her pussy again, wanting so badly to suck her clit *hard*, but knowing it's not quite time yet, gently brushing against it with my lower lip and the tip of my tongue. I slip another finger in, listening to her hard breathing, and then stop everything all together when I hear her groan a little, giggle, and say, 'Guess what he's doing right now?'

My eyes are open because I can't believe what's happening, but then there's a tap on my head and I focus back on giving her what she needs and as she laughs, says, 'God, at *least* two hundred dollars an hour!' I 'm flooded in nervous energy.

'Maybe I can lend him to you,' Sylvia says, laughing again, then moaning quietly in a self-conscious way, lifting her legs a little, her thighs brushing against my ears so that I miss some of the conversation, keeping my hands and tongue and focus on her pussy, thighs, arse.

'But you have to promise to look after him.' I take advantage of the way she lifts her hips to slide a third finger into her pussy and my little finger into her arsehole, wanting this to be perfect for Sylvia, wanting to put on the best performance for Jacqui.

Sylvia's beyond laughing now and kind of breathes amusement at something Jacqui must have said. She whispers before giving in, groaning more naturally and, disappointingly, says, 'I have to go.'

Her phone drops to the bed and she runs her hands through her hair, pulling at it, rocking her hips so that I have to match her movements to keep building her in the right direction and I can tell she's almost there when she starts saying, *'oh shit, oh shit'* in a breathy, high-pitched tone.

I start sucking her clit hard, still flicking my tongue over it, bracing myself for the violence of orgasm when we hear Monica yell out, 'Hey, are you guys up here?'

On reflex, I pull away but Sylvia takes me by the hair and pulls me back in, and after she turns her head towards our open bedroom door, yells, 'Don't come up yet. Stay down there!'

Even with Monica and Doug out there, I somehow maintain my focus on Sylvia. She grips her knees and pulls them up to tilt her pussy and arse further off the bed and, in rolling a little to the side, causes my iPhone cover to flip open only centimetres from my face, revealing that I've somehow failed to notice *four* different notifications.

She's so close to orgasm and has replaced 'oh shit, oh shit' with 'stay there, stay there' because she's crossed over, I recognise it; there's sweet mindlessness in Sylvia's response to what I'm doing, and as I look past my phone to find her face, I realise she's arched up hard. I can only see her exposed belly, her breasts, and hard nipples under her T-shirt.

The ache in my belly and cock and balls is as intense as it's ever been, and at first, there's the instinctive need to reach back, or to grind myself against the bed, but then Sylvia lifts her head from the pillow and I remember that I'm not allowed to touch myself. I understand what it means to be under her spell. I don't want this ache to be relieved.

'Cock,' she says, up on one elbow, teeth still clenching, pointing at my zipper so that I unzip and unbutton and get my pants down mid-thigh, and just being out there, unbound and observed, is enough to flood me with pleasure.

The lust-haze has descended, is thickening, and I'm confused, being torn from Sylvia's needs towards mine so that when she takes a handful of my T-shirt and pulls me onto her, I'm ready to protest and say, 'Let me suck your pussy,' but she has her legs around my waist now. Her hand is a fist, holding my cock against her pussy but only allowing it to penetrate halfway.

She maintains her grip, squeezing the base of my cock tighter and tighter, circling her hips so that her pussy sucks at my cock in a way that burns me out of submission and I've forgotten about her altogether.

I'm fucking as hard and as fast as I can, my hands pushing into the pillow, with my arms locked, keeping my upper body away from the bed so that I can thump my cock through her fist, so that I can fuck that fist out of the way and get the whole length of my cock into the cunt, so that I can force that cunt open and slap my balls against that ass and fill that cunt and find the very end of that cunt. The haze has become a fog so dense, there's no way to see through it and nothing else can exist, not even breath, until a voice I somehow recognise says, 'stop' and then 'get up' and finding me in the fog…Sylvia.

She shifts forward and rides her bum up my squatted thighs and only lets go of my cock so that she can turn her hand over for a better grip, rubbing a little harder, a little faster, a little harder, a little faster, until I'm throwing my head back, eyes closed, covering my face with both hands, hips locked forward at that point of no return. And then, suddenly, she stops rubbing me and all sensation stops.

'Ruined it,' she says.

Sylvia's staring into my eyes with a kind of evil awe, holding the base of my cock, pushing hard into my pubic bone so that I can't move, can't even *thrust*. All orgasmic sensation has ebbed away but I'm amazed to see one thick stream of cum spurting over her belly and pussy, followed by another and then another, so that I'm emptied out but feeling horny as ever, and still under her spell.

'What did you do?' I say, in a kind of whisper, as we both watch her circling the head of my cock around her pussy lips and clit, the rest of my load simply leaking out of me in a way I can only perceive as erotically...*pathetic*.

'You said you wanted to suck my pussy,' she whispers, after shifting her bum away from me, reaching forward to wrap her hands around my neck, dragging me with her as she falls back onto the bed.

I should resist this, is a thought, as she forces my head between her thighs, *I should protest*, is another, but the thought that trumps both of them is this one – *those are online thoughts, not offline thoughts.*

This is forbidden, and *so* dirty, and not what I'm supposed to do, and maybe that's why I'm shaking all over and consumed by newness and confusion and shame, as if I'm having sex for the very first time.

Sylvia's so wet with her cum and mine that I slide my little finger into her arsehole easily, and then another as I flatten my tongue and lick along both fingers, over her pussy opening, dipping in a little, flicking at the end of her clit, before starting at my fingers again to gather the taste of us – the two of us together – from her left labia, and then her right labia, and I think I know where she's going with this, I think I know what fantasy she's losing herself in, I think I know what she's been thinking about and planning, for maybe *months* now. And right now, as I take in as much of her pussy as I can, sucking hard and sliding my lips together until they're closed over, until my mouth is full enough that I have to swallow *twice*, I'm almost certain I can do it for her.

I'm holding my hand still against her just as she did to me, but there'd be no way to prevent her orgasm, even if I wanted to, because she's forced two fingers and most of my thumb into her pussy just by thrusting up and down and grinding into me and I'm clamped between her thighs doing my best to keep my mouth over her clit, sucking, flicking, just as she likes it, right to the very end, and I can't hear much, can't even open my eyes, am actually worried I might run out of breath, swimming in euphoria, aware in such a joyous, unrestricted way, that this kind of Sylvia – a kind of *violence* – is the kind I really need, and with my fingers inside her, while waiting for the shuddering to subside, , I'm almost more curious than horny about this thing that's happening to me, this thing that almost seems inevitable, which began with the sharing of the BBC pic, or maybe right back to when the surveillance teddy gave Sylvia the opportunity to observe me in my natural habitat away from the gaze of others. And I'm only released from this reverie when she puts her hands on my face and guides it to hers.

She kisses me, sucks softly on my bottom lip, says, 'Fuck you, *Multi-Mum*. I'm the only one who can call Joel a pervert,' and after kissing again, we become aware of a voice that seems to be coming from a distance but that I track to Sylvia's phone, which is lying on the pillow next to her.

'Shit!' Sylvia picks up her phone, laugh-squealing, and because I'm face to face with her, I can hear that it's Jacqui.

'Oh my God. He just *has* to open a shop,' Jacqui says.

'A shop?' I say, querying eyes on Sylvia, and I can tell by the way she's grimacing and smiling at the same time that she wants to relax and enjoy herself but is worried about my reaction to this. 'What shop?'

When it becomes clear that the laughter on the other end of the phone belongs to more than just one woman, a charge of shame slash mortification slash BBC-Facebook-sharing *hysteria* combines with my torrential lust to mute me, so that I'm just staring at Sylvia, wide-eyed; surprised emoticon.

'Okay, I'll let you guys get back to it,' Jacqui says, sing-song. 'See you tomorrow, hun,' and then, a little breezy. 'Bye, Joel...'

Sylvia drops the phone and looks at me, eyebrows raised.

'Oops?' I say, beating her to it.

She runs her fingers up my back, and as she bites her lip like that – crazy sexy – her expression softens. 'That was an honest accident. I thought I'd ended the call. But you don't have to worry...'

The muffled sound of my phone ringing and vibrating makes her jump a little, because she's lying on it, and I'm up on my knees as she fishes it out from under her ass. 'Oh, no,' she says.

'Oh, no,' I say, snatching it from her. The cover's all wet and so I get the phone out of it as fast I can, relieved from a mild panic when I see that it's still working properly, that I won't have to soak it in a bowl of rice and wait twenty-four hours to get online.

Sylvia hits me in the chest and swings her leg past me, and as I'm opening Facebook to see that my event post has already received many comments, 42 Likes, and 4 Shares, she says, 'I think Monica and Doug are out there.'

THE BEST ENGAGEMENT

87:14:14

I'm up on my feet, pulling my pants up, wiping my face and hands and iPhone cover with yesterday's T-shirt before I realise something that stops me dead. Our bedroom door, which was open before, is now eerily closed, and suddenly, the shame and the mortification are winning.

Sylvia's straightening out her T-shirt and shorts and as I throw my T-shirt to the laundry basket and notice the wet patch on the doona, she mouths, 'Are they out there?' while pointing at the door.

'Fold the doona over,' I say, opening the door and poking my head out to see Monica emerging from the stairs, with Doug just behind her carrying his heavy suitcase.

'Oh, hey,' Monica says. 'We're just moving Doug's things into the room next to Dylan's.'

'That's a good room,' I say, stupidly, eyes down, tapping the password into my coverless phone, opening settings as if I have an important task to perform.

Doug says, 'Awesome house, Joel', and even though I wait to look up until they've passed by, I can still tell that he's beaming.

'Did they see?' Sylvia whispers, grimacing.

My hands rise a little and fall to my sides and I'm holding my breath listening to the laughter coming down the hall, searching for relief in how unaffected it sounds, but I still jump a little and sit next to Sylvia when Monica knocks on the wall in the hallway outside our room.

'Come in' Sylvia says.

Monica walks in, says 'Hi,' hands behind her, leaning into the wall, and after Sylvia says 'Hi' with a little *fake*-laugh, I hold up my hand and wiggle my fingers for some reason, *over*-smiling. Then, as we create a square-ish cone of silence, Doug also putting his hands behind him to lean in against the wall – so that he and Monica are standing beside each other as if they've been summoned into the principal's office – Sylvia straightens out her legs, leans forward as if she's doing a hamstring stretch, lifts her hands, slaps her knees, says, 'So…did you see?'

The answer is right there, before Monica says anything, in the way Doug starts snorting through his nose, trying not to laugh.

'Just a little bit,' Monica says, without a hint of embarrassment, holding a forefinger and thumb about four centimetres apart.

'I didn't hear anything,' I say, as Sylvia props her head in her hands, covering her mouth and nose, her cheeks flushed. 'I didn't even see the door close.'

'You couldn't have seen or heard anything from where you were,' Monica says, and as I get another phone call that I decide not to answer – the third one from Jen in the past hour – Doug really lets go, laughing and smacking his hands together, and I'm not really so surprised, with all that's happened to me, that it's Sylvia who's seeming the most mortified by this.

'Look, Sylvia!' I say, taking her by the shoulder and pulling her into me. 'Doug's only been here for five minutes and he's already *lol-ing.*'

'Don't worry,' Doug says, gaining control of himself. 'I toured with a male dance group. I've seen some crazy stuff. You guys are so awesome…'

'You guys are so…fucking hot,' Monica says, shaking her head as if she's just run into a Kardashian. 'You're so…*cute.* You should pose for Hell Pa, for the exhibition.'

My phone appears before me at the mention of the exhibition, and as I'm clipping it back into the cover, the whole house appears before me and it occurs to me that it doesn't feel like such a monstrosity to me anymore – it feels about right, we've just about filled every room so that it has energy, it feels alive. 'That's actually a pretty good idea, Monica. Hell Pa should paint a portrait of *everyone* in the house,' I say, which triggers my memory of Taylor, so that I stand up, swipe away a Twitter notification I don't even read, and say to Sylvia, 'There's a woman downstairs who's moving in with us.' I'm smiling a little at the strangeness I'm about to deliver. 'Her name's Taylor. She's a transgender person…and has a penis.'

'Oh,' Sylvia says, lifting her head, pleased suddenly. 'She's here already?'

'You know about her?' I say, as I Like several comments on my event post, all of which are very positive.

'Of course, I found her on Craigslist.'

'Hell Pa's doing her portrait,' I say, so surprised that it sounds like I'm asking a question. 'For the exhibition.'

When she sneaks a laugh, I turn to Doug and Monica who are both smiling, in a knowing way, and I'm locked in on Doug, thinking *how the fuck do you seem to know what's going on around here* when Sylvia says, 'She's not just here for the portrait, Joel,' and I'm almost getting it, I've just about got it, until a notification from Doug's phone distracts me, at the same time a voice from down stairs – Diana's – calls out.

'Up here, Mum.'

Sylvia stands up, kisses me on the cheek, and after some distinctly mother-in-law-ish pitter-pattering of feet on the carpeted stairs, a large, square screen print of a city park bench surrounded by trees, back-dropped by a city landscape, comes through the door, with Diana right behind.

'I think this is going to be perfect for the wall adjacent to the front door,' she says, glancing at all of us with only a hint of confusion. 'People will walk past the Japanese maples, to the industrial-*ness* of the building and then see nature and civilisation combined in this painting. It will give an immediate sense of…um—'

'A kind of warmth,' I say, shrugging, smiling because this is like…escalating. 'I *love* the venue you chose for the exhibition, Diana,' I say, after everyone *loves* the screen print enthusiastically. 'I really *love* the venue.'

When Doug asks what the venue looks like, Diana, Monica, and I lift our phones simultaneously to retrieve a photo. Diana laughs and apologises, and Monica laughs and apologises, and because I was just Liking comments on the event post, I scroll back to the picture and hand it over to Doug.

'This is the Facebook event I've created for the exhibition,' I say. 'Do you think you could share it on your Facebook page?'

'Of course,' Doug says, super enthusiastic as usual, using his finger and thumb to enlarge the photo. 'Wow. Awesome stage.'

'We can get the keys tomorrow,' Diana says. 'I've booked it for a whole week.'

Monica looks over Doug's shoulder and says, 'I'll share it on my Facebook page, as well.'

'What's your Facebook page?' I ask.

'*Moments with Monica*,' she says. 'It's mostly quotes I find…and some crafty things.'

'How many Likers do you have?' I ask.

'Only about seven thousand,' she says. 'But I've got way more followers on Pinterest. Over twenty thousand.'

'Holy *shit*!' I say, as Doug hands back my iPhone so that he can focus back on *his* iPhone and then Sylvia's standing next to me, flipping the cover on *her* iPhone, and I'm forced to acknowledge something wonderful: we are a circle of phones in the main bedroom, and everyone is focused together on the one thing.

When Diana says, 'I'll share it, as well,' I point at her dramatically and say, 'You do *not* have a Facebook page,' and then, because I start laughing in such an hysterical fashion after she says, 'Only a *personal* page,' everyone *else* starts laughing, and I imagine a camera pulling away from us, circling above and rising towards the sky.

'Don't share anything yet,' I say, holding my hand out. 'Let's wait until tonight and share it all together. I always get the best online engagement after 8pm.'

'Yeah, me, too,' Monica says.

'Good idea,' Sylvia says, elbowing me. 'It'll give me time to fix your event description.'

'Hey,' Doug says. 'What if I dance?'

'What?' I say, reaching out, slapping the back of my hand against Sylvia's stomach, as if I'm stopping a child from running onto a busy road.

'I could really *own* that stage, man…even use a lot of the hall…depending on the size of the crowd.'

'Front row seats!' Diana says, raising her hand.

'I'll just need some props,' he says, as mine and Sylvia's hands – which are very sticky – entwine, and I feel like I've already defeated *Multi-Mum*.

Her crusade against me is over before it's begun. I can see her standing under a small square of tarp which is propped up by four gangly tent poles and her small army – Simeon the puppet and those plasticky others – are huddling underneath it holding cold sausages and stale bread, fuelled by nothing more than blind hope as a torrential rain pours, running off the tarp in long lines to form a kind of watery prison. It's so clear in my mind that it's as if I've already Instagrammed it.

'Please tell me you'll do the "Pony" routine,' I say, barely a whisper.

'I'll do the "Pony" routine,' Doug says, pausing as Sylvia actually says, 'Squee' without any real surprise, as if she was expecting this, before he adds, 'If you do it with me…'

He's caught me off guard, but I can't respond anyway, because Dylan's scream, 'Daddy!' rises up to the first floor to drape me in a cold dread, and although we all react at the same time, I'm the first person to burst into the hallway to his rescue.

CAPTURED

Dylan yells 'Daddy!' again and I'm drawn forward by the apparent need in his tone and propelled even faster by the sounds of hands and shoulders banging against the walls and sliding down the railing behind me and I'm just about terrified when I hear Diana scream, 'Oh, no!' as I leap over the last step and grip the door frame, swinging myself into the art studio to see Dylan standing next to Hell Pa. They're both standing in front of easels wearing smocks, holding paintbrushes, perfectly okay, with Taylor just behind them in a dressing gown.

Doug bumps up against me for the second time since he moved in and says, 'Is everything okay?' as Sylvia rushes past and falls to her knees, taking Dylan by the shoulders.

'He's okay,' Hell Pa says, bewildered. 'He just wants to show you a painting.'

'I painted Taylor,' Dylan says. 'Like Hell Pa.'

'It sounded like you were freaking dying,' Sylvia says, hand on her heart. 'God.'

'I was tickling him,' Taylor says, wiggling her fingers at Sylvia, whispering sorry, and while they're going through their 'oohs!' and 'ahhs!' and 'great to finally meet you!'s, I stand between the canvases and let my gaze drift over Dylan's painting – a portrait of Taylor's face.

Hell Pa's painting is a surreal full body portrait. Taylor's penis curls around her waist twice and she's cradling the head – which has transformed into the shape of a baby – in her arms, breastfeeding it.

After coming to the conclusion very quickly that both paintings are equal in terms of mastery; they are both just, really, *shit* paintings, and with my heart rate returning to normal, I feel a suspended kind of joy for Dylan because this is still *way* better than any of the artwork he brings home from school. Here we are, in a less structured environment, and he's already shown that he's as talented as Hell Pa, a painter who's skilled enough to have more Likers on Facebook than me.

'These paintings are very good,' I say, squeezing Dylan's shoulders. 'But I think yours is *way* better.'

'Aww,' Taylor says. 'I think Hell Pa's painting is good, as well.'

'You do?' I say, looking over my shoulder to see Taylor pointing at Dad, mouthing *No* and shaking her head as if she's tasted something sour.

'I really do,' she says, reaching out, rubbing his back.

Diana appears at the door holding up the screen print to reveal a massive hole in the middle of it and when Doug says, 'Oh, no,' and Monica says, 'Oh, that's a shame,' Diana laughs at herself, says, 'I stood on it,' and I have this feeling that my life is out of my hands, that maybe it always has been. The small space I occupy in the world is inside a petri dish filled with water and sand and there's a scientist tipping it back and forth, from one end to the other, swirling it round and round in circles, just to see what happens.

I open my Sonos app to get some music going and it's as the slow spacey intro to Single Pill's "I Can't Feel My Face" begins to build in several rooms around the house that Diana leans into the hallway, says, 'There's someone at the door.'

We all stop collectively as a panicky, muffled voice reaches us.

'Who is it?' I say, as the scientist tips the dish one way and then the other and then swirls everything around with the end of her little finger.

I'm pushing past Doug as he picks up Dylan and turns him upside down and the music sounds out a little more loudly than I'd anticipated, creating a kind of urgency. I rush by Diana and open the front door to see Jen wearing a beige tracksuit and a studded dog collar, yell-crying, '*Multi-Mum*'s just a self-centred lying *bitch!*' to a woman in a long, black, tight-fitting dress, heavy make-up, hair in a bun, with two men behind her, one with a large camera on his shoulder, the other holding a big furry microphone above Jen's head.

'It's *The Daily Events*', Jen says, pulling Audrey behind her and hightailing it up the hallway.

When I turn around to track her progress, I see that everyone else is behind me and because they look just as stunned as I do, I start running as fast as I can as well, but in the opposite direction for some reason, out the front door, past the woman in the black dress and the cameraman and the furry microphone and leaping over the flower bed.

'Joel Anstey?' the woman yells, clip-clopping after me in her fancy shoes. 'Why do you think it's okay to harass a single mother with pornographic photos?'

Up ahead is a house I've walked past many times and in the front yard right against a wire mesh fence is a hip-high bottlebrush shaped into a long rectangle and I feel instinctively that it's the perfect place to hide behind and small enough that I can jump over it without too much difficulty. But I'm wrong on both counts because as I attempt a kind of Fosbury Flop, my hands scrape the flat surface of the bottlebrush, tearing my phone from my grip as I tumble through the air and onto the sopping lawn with such force that all the wind is knocked out of me.

The pain is almost blinding and as I'm trying to take a breath, commando-crawling, scanning the garden bed for my phone, the huge camera peers over the bottlebrush like an alien about to eat me.

I can see my pathetic form in its lens; the circular mechanisms behind it making tiny adjustments to focus, capturing me as the furry microphone appears alongside it, followed by another smaller black microphone, followed by the face of the woman in the black dress. 'Do you think it's okay to assault school teachers, Mr. Anstey? Do you think it's okay to terrorise children?'

I manage to raise myself to my hands and knees after finally taking in enough air to quell the dull pain in my lungs and there's my phone, trapped in the very middle of the bottlebrush, the cover spread open, several missed notifications visible on the screen.

The woman is still asking questions and the camera's still leering in, trying to eat me, and the first thing I think of after retrieving my phone – my forearms bleeding from several long scratches – is the smugly smiling *Multi-Mum* and then, strangely, as I start growling with the effort of attempting to strangle the furry microphone away from the man who's holding it, Lindsay Lohan sitting in a court room with F.U. painted on her fingernails.

'Let the microphone go, Mr. Anstey,' the woman's yelling. 'What are you ashamed of? What are you ashamed of?'

I only release the microphone when I hear Sylvia yell out, 'Joel!' and look up to see her running down the footpath with Doug and Taylor. Taylor's still wearing the dressing gown and holding her iPhone out, obviously recording.

The cameraman's backed away to capture the whole scene. The woman in the black dress tells Taylor to stop recording as Doug and Sylvia run into the front yard to help me off my knees. The mindless panic that caused me to run in the first place seems to fizzle, leaving only anger. I feel myself eternally indebted to Taylor when she says, 'I'll put my camera down if you put *your* camera down,' even though I know it will achieve nothing.

'Don't worry about it, Joel,' Sylvia says, wrapping her arms around my waist, squeezing her body against mine, ignoring the camera. 'Let's just invite them in. It's just stupid tabloid TV. Let's have fun with it. It'll be great advertisement for the exhibition.'

I can see Doug talking to the reporter woman and she's shaking her head a little, smiling, and Taylor's walking a circle even wider than the cameraman, holding her phone between the thumb and forefingers of both hands, lips pursed, serious, and I become aware of the rain falling, of how wet I am, the tiny flimsy pair of shorts and T-shirt that Sylvia's wearing.

'We'll be on the TV,' I whisper, focused back on her. 'What about your job? Francis will fire you.'

'No,' she says, taking my hand. 'Don't worry about that. He can't ever fire me.'

'Why not?'

'Come on,' she says, walking me towards the gates. 'It'll be great advertisement for the exhibition. And you'll get heaps of Likes.'

**Thanks for reading Some Kind of Superstar
Series One, Episode Three.**

Episodes Four and Five are now available on Amazon at
these links:

Episode Four: http://myBook.to/SKSSS1E4

Episode Five: http://myBook.to/SKSSS1E5

About the Author

C.A. Greagen's humorous and moving memoir Reservoir Dad was published with Random House after his popular blog won the Australian Writers' Centre 'Personal Blog Award' 2013. Truce Films are currently in the process of adapting the book to a feature length film.

Connect with C.A. Greagen

Website:

www.cagreagen.com

Social Networks

Twitter: https://twitter.com/ReservoirDad

Facebook: http://www.facebook.com/ReservoirDad

Instagram: https://www.instagram.com/c.a.greagen

CONTENTS

1.   Doctors (Sonnet 1401)

Doctor Not Butcher
(Medical Anthem Sonnet, 1401)

We are the Doctors,
Our worship is to the ailing.
We don't bow to politicians,
Nor to bureaucratic bullying.

Service to the sick
is service to the divine.
There is no greater divinity,
than being a human lifeline.

We don't recognize borders,
We don't recognize states.
Patientcare is our national anthem,
Reward of medicine is smiling patients.

Dead doctor postpones death,
Living doctor improves life.
While butcher doctors monetize malady,
To empower life, real doctors strive.

Note: Medicine means Mercy - Empathy - Dare - Integrity - Care - Ingenuity - Nobility - and Ethics, or it can mean Mechanical, Egotistical, Dehumanizing, Indifferent, Cold, Insensitive, Nincompoop Elitist. You decide what you practice, and your decision will determine what you are - a doctor or a butcher! Just remember one thing - the only permanence we have is each other.

2.   Healers (Sonnet 1402 - 1404)

Smile Before Pills (Sonnet 1402)

The only permanence we have is each other,
The only paradise we have is each other.
Heaven is as real as we are to each other,
Most potent medicine we have is each other.

One moment of love is time eternal,
100 years of hate are but ghost of wild past.
One rebellion of love is destiny in making,
100 rituals of hate are just monkeys' mass.

A smile works faster than a pill,
both metaphorically and physiologically.
Pills take hours to reach your bloodstream, while
a smile triggers instant release of neurochemicals,
which alleviates pain and facilitates immunity.

Sure, pills and prescriptions are a scientific boon,
They achieve wonders where organic powers fall short.
Yet, there is no prescription for a mannerless medico,
There is no pharmaceutical cure for a medical upstart.

Sonnet 1403

Entire world is a church,
The innocents are our deities.
Helping the helpless is divine service,
In their smile unfolds heavenly peace.

Above everything kindness is real,
Save kindness all is unspiritual.
Above all else people are real,
There ain't no paradise but people.

Not all are doctors, but healers we all,
Healing the ailing we redeem divinity.
We don't need some fictitious magic,
Miracle unfolds through magnanimity.

Entire world is church-n-mosque,
Folks forsaken are our deity.
Above all else humans are true,
Ain't no divinity but humanity.

Sonnet 1404

Divide and divine
can never go together,
Hate and human
can never go together.

Conscience and conspiracy
can never go together,
Reason and rigidity
can never go together.

United we are heroes,
divided we are ashes.
United we are alive,
divided we are dead.

Inclusivity empowers integrity,
Integrity empowers character.
Character empowers civilization,
Civilization empowers inclusivity.

3. Illumination (Sonnet 1405 - 1407)

Sonnet 1405

Inclusion is illumination,
Segregation is degeneration.
Prejudice is utter unpiety,
No matter the indoctrination.

Humanity is divinity,
Divinity is poetry.
Poetry is illumination,
Illumination is sanity.

Illumination ain't supernatural,
There is no magical vibration.
Past old and modern superstition,
Mind ushers into realization.

True giants live past superstition,
They got no use for comforting lies.
We have too many real life issues
to waste our force of life on lies.

The Carnivore (Sonnet 1406)

Be a gentle giant like the elephant,
not an opportunistic carnivore like the wolf.
The elephant doesn't harm anyone
to prove its greatness, while the wolf
doesn't think twice to devour another wolf.

Greatness unfolds through gentleness,
Illumination unfolds through expansion.
Coldness is the mark of cowardly animal,
Cruelty is cover for beastly degeneration.

Worst of all carnivores are the humans,
There is no end to their appetite.
Animals no longer partake once they are full,
While human greed knows no sane height.

More clothes, more cars, more cash,
Just how much will you consider enough!
Till you put a cork on cocky abundance,
Not felicity but disparity wreaks havoc.

Savagest carnivore of all is the human.
Uncorked materialism is new cannibalism.

Note: If I ask - are you an ordinary person - all the
ordinary people will promptly say, they are not -

while only the few extraordinary souls will say, they are quite ordinary. You see, true greatness doesn't disconnect you from the ordinary people, it only makes you more ordinary - more ordinarily conscious, more ordinarily conscientious, more ordinarily responsible. In fact, the more extraordinary you are, the more ordinary you feel. And only with such existential ordinariness shall we change the world, not with empty, snobbish extraordinariness. So I ask again - I am very much ordinary - are you?

Sonnet 1407

My sufiness doesn't come from Koran,
My advaitaness doesn't come from Vedanta.
My humanism doesn't come from science,
Everything I am comes from my conscience.

My goodness doesn't come from God,
God's goodness comes from me.
God and I are not two, but one,
God and I are one existentiality.

Fact of the matter is that,
Question of God is irrelevant.
Focus on acts of kindness instead,
You'll be the epitome of godliness.

Mark you, I ain't glorifying facts -
All I ask is, you attend to ascension.
Beyond all crucifix and calculus,

Love is the only cosmic education.

Buluşalım (Şiir)

Dilin ve dinin ötesinde bir yer var,
orada buluşacağım seninle.
Vatanın ve varoluşun ötesinde gel,
buluşalım, artık bekleme.
Korkunun ve köktenciliğin ötesinde,
Hoşgörüsüzlüğün ve haksızlığın ötesinde,
Acımasızlığın ve amaçsızlığın ötesinde,
İlgisizliğin ve umutsuzluğun ötesinde,
bir yer var, orada buluşacağım seninle.
Zekânın ve cehaletin ötesinde,
Bir gün gel, artık bekletme.

4.   Insight (Sonnet 1408 - 1410)

They ask me, do I ever worry about losing my magic? I tell them, my only worry is that, some day I might lose the morale that makes the magic possible. I pour magic because my mind is ablaze - the day the fire goes out, so does my magic.

Sonnet 1408

Ain't no rest for the reformer,
no matter the legacy I leave behind.
Point of it all is to stir up vigor,
that ends all feelings unkind.

Morale makes the magic possible,
Where there's morale, there's magic.
Unyielding morale is my gift to thee,
Use it wisely for collective uplift.

The more I write,
the more I realize,
I've written nothing.
The more I understand,
the more I realize,
I understand nothing.

Sonnet 1409

Intelligence makes you smug,
Understanding makes you humble.
To know what you know is knowledge,
To know what you don't is wisdom.

I am wise because I am an idiot,
I am an idiot because I am wise.
My insight isn't rooted in intelligence,
My insight is rooted in humankind.

Insight and intelligence are not the same,
Insight often demands omission of intelligence.
If you don't know the right place for intelligence,
Not an insightful human, you're just a clever ape.

Insight makes you absolutely free
from the chains of both comforting fiction
and narcissistic intelligence.
So long as you are slave to either,
you are anything but a sapiens.

Sapiens (Sonnet 1410)

Sapiens is a promise
to stand grounded in people,
Sapiens is a duty
to stand firm on principle.

Sapiens is an alarm
to wake up from apathy,
Sapiens is mindful revolt
against inherited atrocity.

Sapiens is rightful rebellion
against dehumanizing intellect,
Sapiens is sentient uproar
against puritanism boneheaded.

Sapiens is the saintly answer
to the clarion call of life,
True sapiens is saintly sapiens,
all else is desecration of life.

5.   Fruitcake (Sonnet 1411 - 1413)

Sonnet 1411

I am most content when I am writing as a sufi,
Writing as humanitarian takes excruciating toll.
That's why I find it sustainable to switch spirits,
Between dervish, humanitarian and nondual roles.

Right now I speak to you as sufi,
All I do is draw from my wounds.
Afterwards I gotta set my blood on fire,
World War Human unfolds through fiery truth.

One shoe does not fit all feet,
One raw idea doesn't answer all problems.
Answer must be molded compatible with context,
Contextless answer creates only more problems.

That is why I am sufi where sufi is needed,
Then a humanitarian when that's what's needed.
The spirit takes many forms across cultures,
Be love and see love, for love is always needed.

Sonnet 1412

The Catholic Church is one of the
ghastliest invading forces in history,
alongside the British, French and Spaniards.
But don't confuse the Vatican with Jesus -
Jesus was rejuvenation, Vatican, disaster.

Jesus was a spirit of love and light,
the answer of his time to bigotry.
Yet he ended up as institutional excuse
in new exploits of counterfeit piety.

You say, Jesus died for your sins,
Yet you killed more people in his name.
Vatican is the epitome of unholiness,
Slaves to Vatican are clinically insane.

Not just Vatican, but every religious
institution is a septic tank of prejudice.
Till you cut ties to all authoritarianism,
you'll never sense the spark of holiness.

Sonnet 1413

To be whole
or be in hole,
that is the question.
To be amiable
or be tamable,
that is the question.

To click or not to click,
that's the trillion dollar
mental health question.
To scroll or not to scroll,
that's the zillion dollar
mindfulness question.

To be visionbound
or be biasbound,
that is the question.
To be heartbound
or be hatebound,
that is the question.

To sow the seeds of fruit
or to be the fruitcake,
that is the question.
Wholeness bears fruits of life,
Holeness causes castration.

6.   Lightning (Sonnet 1414 - 1416)

Sonnet 1414

I am not a capitalist,
I am not a communist,
I am not a socialist,
I am not a traditionalist.

A puerile, clinically sectarian species
like yours cannot fathom what I am.
Does that mean, I am not the same
species as you! Sure, I am -

but from a different dimension -
a different dimension in time -
a different dimension in mind -

where intellect is only a tool, not torture -
where faith is only a choice, not compulsion -
where money is only a means, not master -
where oneness is fundamental, not fiction.

Sonnet 1415

I stand for virtues, not ideologies
claiming to have codified those virtues.
I stand for valor, not traditions
claiming to have a franchise over valor.

I stand for honor, not slavery
claiming to be the sign of honor.
I stand for conscience, not ignorance
claiming to be the bearer of conscience.

I stand for awakening, not slumber
claiming to symbolize higher awakening.
I stand for insight, not blindness
claiming to be the deliverer of sight.

I stand for humanity, not for nations
claiming to contain the best of humanity.
I stand for life, not for labels
claiming to know what's best for everybody.

Divine Lightning
(Sonnet 1416)

We are the rivers,
We are the confluence.
We are the zenith,
We are the mountains.

We are the climber,
We are the climb.
We are the clock,
We are the time.

We are the memory,
We are the moments.
We are living piety,
We are the prophets.

We are the God,
We are the Goblins.
Amidst fanatic foolery
We are divine lightning.

7.   Inoculation (Sonnet 1417 - 1419)

Tanrı'dan Şiir Mektubu

Bazıları bana Tanrı diyor,
Bazıları diyor "Bhagvan".
Bazıları "Lord God" diyor,
Ama ben aslında insan.

Beni camide değil,
insanların içinde ara.
Cami Tanrısız olabilir,
ama Tanrı insansız olamaz.

Laiklik yani dini terk etmek değil,
Laiklik yani, köktenciliğe karşı aşılamak.
Kör inanca kafa gömmek kutsallık değil,
İlahiyat yani inancın ötesinde insana sarılmak.

Her şeyin üstünde insan gerçek,
İnsanın üstünde hiçbir şey yok.
Tanrılık ve İnsanlık aynı şey,
İnsanlıktan başka tanrılık yok.

Letter from God
(An Autobiographical Sonnet, 1417)

Some people chant Bismillah,
Some people chant Bhagvan.
Some people call me Lord God,
I'm actually very much human.

Seek me in church and temple,
I shall elude you for time eternal.
All churches are without God,
But God cannot be without human.

Above all hagiographies, human is real,
There's nothing more divine than human.
Godliness unfolds only through humanness,
Only sin in the world is the sin of division.

Secularism is not a rejection of religion,
secularism is inoculation against fundamentalism.
Religion is not the search for a mythical deity,
but the realization of oneness within every human.

Sonnet 1418

Secularism is not a rejection of religion,
secularism is inoculation against fundamentalism.
Religion is not the search for a mythical deity,
but the realization of love within the human.

However, now let's get beyond the ism,
Let's leave all terminologies behind.
Forget secularism, just foster oneness,
That is existence, most divine kind.

Don't pay too much attention to terms,
Secularism, Humanism and so on.
Main thing is your behavior,
Rest is shallow speculation.

Hence, ardent critics of religion
are just as animal as fundamentalists.
The goal is to open our heart to all,
not just to fancy intellectualists.

Sonnet 1419

When things go wrong,
intellectuals are the first to scarper,
because it's easier to find flaws
than to be the problem solver.

During the first year I tried to write like
an intellectual, until I realized, that's not me.
So I abandoned the intellectual facade,
and became unapologetically human in my writing,
and I haven't looked back since.

The tone of 'In Search of Divinity' was so different
that I even thought of publishing by a pseudonym.
Today I am glad that I did not change my name,
for the different new tone was the true voice of mine.

Monkey see, monkey imitate -
Human challenge is to find yourself.
Once you do, that's when you start to glow,
Synthetic sparklers only drag you to descent.

8.   Grownup (Sonnet 1420 - 1422)

Sonnet 1420

Intellect used as an intellectual
diminishes your humanity,
Intellect used as a human
enhances your humanity.

Faith used as a believer
diminishes your humanity,
Faith used as a human
enhances your humanity.

The moment an identity becomes more important
than your humanity, you become less human.
Now you might argue, isn't humanity an identity!
Humanity isn't identity, humanity is existence.

Anything sectarian is an impediment to humanity.
Be whatever you like, but first belong to humanity.

Sonnet 1421

Humanity is not given,
Humanity is a choice.
Every moment you're given to choose,
humanity over sectarian allegiance.

Integrity is not fed,
Integrity is fostered.
Honor is not inherited,
Honor is earned.

Every moment is moment of truth,
that unveils your worth as a human.
Human worth is determined by behavior,
not whether you believe in fiction.

Belief defines a child,
Behavior defines a grownup.
Intellectual or religious doesn't matter,
What matters is how you treat others.

Sonnet 1422

Comic book fans
come in many forms -
Some attend comicon,
Some visit the vatican,
Some visit vrindavan.

Some bury head in the bible,
Some bury head in das kapital.
When pages of books are
prioritized over humanity,
world gets infested with sheeple.

Mind begins in the wake of chains,
Life begins in the wake of sect.
A hundred hajj won't make you holy,
If your heart is ever cold and dead.

58

9. Lifting (Sonnet 1423 - 1425)

Every Religion is Right Religion
(Unscriptured Holiness Sonnet, 1423)

Islam* is not the right religion, *peace is.
Christianity** is no right religion, **kindness is.
Judaism is not the right religion, equality is.
Sanatana isn't right religion, nonsectarianism is.

All scriptures are blasphemy, when peddled
as exclusive, infallible handbook to divinity.
Literature that demands rejection of backbone,
is a lot of things but not material of sanctity.

Every religion is right religion, or none are;
Claiming exclusive rightness all breed cowards.
Every faith is an attempt at divine, or none are;
Claiming monopoly of truth faith forfeits regard.

By saying your religion is the only right religion,
you only prove, your religion is the wrong religion.
Religion as an excuse for separation is always wrong,
till you transcend religion, all faith is delusion.

Sonnet 1424

An evening spent lifting your neighborhood
is far holier than an audience with the pope.
Pope's holiness comes from your belief,
Your holiness comes from your action.

Jesus and pope are not the same,
Jesus was love, pope is a position
cashing in on that love.
The same is true for every religious
institution, though no other institution
is as extravagant as the vatican.

Holiness begins with love,
Love begins with freedom.
Love that comes with bible attached,
is not love, but holy degeneration.

Mind begins in the wake of chains,
Life begins at the wake of sect.
Vaticans rise and vaticans fall,
Only thing timeless is heart without sect.

Sonnet 1425

Naskar nation - integration.
Naskar reason - assimilation.
Naskar vision - invigoration.
Naskar mission - unification.

Neither nearsighted nor farsighted,
I am simply insighted.
Neither tribal, nor global,
I'm simply mind ignited.

Time is born of awareness,
Unawareness just ruins time.
If you want time, be aware -
Fabric of time is born of mind.

Awareness begets contentment,
Awareness begets time.
The unaware is cruel,
while the aware is kind.

64

10. Phone (Sonnet 1426 - 1428)

Grownup Happiness
(The Sonnet, 1426)

I don't do Netflix,
I don't binge for adrenaline.
I find it far more soothing to
listen to old BBC radio shows
while I do my writing.

Happiness is not a matter of exhilaration,
Happiness is a matter of moderation.
Just because all the monkeys are partying,
doesn't mean you gotta give submission.

So I say, get your priorities straight,
Happiness will take care of itself.
If you don't know to draw your own lines,
That's not freedom, but apish descent.

I don't scroll till I pass out,
I don't drink till I feel sick.
Happiness means happy-in-less,
Trends don't bring you peace.

Sonnet 1427

If you use social media,
don't ask for privacy.
If you want privacy,
don't use social media.

App after app, post after post,
Your phone becomes an apparatus of sickness.
Learn to prioritize people over phone,
That's the sustainable road to happiness.

You don't need to abandon your phone,
Every era has its basic requirements.
But remember just one little thing,
Never let gadgets take over awareness.

People before phone,
Society before technology.
If you don't get this,
I wish you a nice tech-slavery.

Sonnet 1428

When your first thought
of the day is one person,
When last thought before
sleep is one person,

When their growth
expands your soul,
When their smile
makes your face glow,

When their tears wreak
havoc in your heart,
When their achievements
brighten your world,

That, my friend, is intimacy in action -
That's when two become one.

11. Dumped (Sonnet 1429 - 1431)

72

One and A Half Ex
(Sonnet 1429)

Once upon a time by the Bay of Bengal,
a naive tiger fell for a vain sheep.
The sheep had him eating out of her hand,
only to discard him for another sheep.

The tiger's world was turned upside down,
abandoning home-n-uni he set out as monk.
Then one afternoon underneath the tree,
the monk awakened to prophetic dimension.

The saintly tiger then returned home,
Lo, commenced his sleepless self-education!
He had already mastered all divine sight,
Now he needed to muster a scientific arsenal.

Sonnet 1430

During his making he met a Balkan xena,
she was everything he could ever dream of.
But the tiger still had plenty struggle ahead,
even for the perfect partner it was too much.

She had a beautiful heart which grew weary,
waiting for a giant with the world on shoulder.
The first whole love of the tiger came to halt,
after four magical years of timeless forever.

Though devastated, unable to think-n-work,
this time this was no longer a naive tiger.
Gloom galvanizes conviction invincible,
Shattered heart makes shade for the world.

Yeşil Gözler
(Balkan Şiir)

Bazen Kara Sevda'da yaşıyormuşum gibi geliyor,
Pernik'teki o yeşil gözler Nihan'a benziyor.

Beş yılı birlikte geçirdikten sonra karar verdin,
ben sana layık değildim, çünkü henüz yoktu para.
Yaraları bir kenara bırakıp mücadeleye devam ettim,
Bugün sen bana layık değilsin, diyorum ben sana.

Sana en çok ihtiyacım olduğu anda sen vazgeçtin,
Ama yine de bu gerçek aşık sana beddua etmiyo.
Sevgili değil artık, insan olarak destek olacağım,
Kendine iyi bak - kiminle olursan ol mutlu ol!

Dünyadaki bütün aşıklara diyorum,
eğer seviyorsan kendini kaybederek sev.
Binlerce kez ihanete uğra, ayıp değil,
ama asla kimseye beddua etme.

Sonnet 1431

Put your heart out there trampling caution.
Don't be afraid, just put it out there.
If it's rescued, you receive love.
If it's refused, you receive valor.

I speak to all the lovers of the world,
If you wanna love, do so obliterating the self.
Be shattered to a thousand pieces - ain't a shame!
But to another's joy never be an impediment.

There's no glory in dumping the other first,
Any self-obsessed animal can do that.
Be a human lover and stand boldly vulnerable,
Better be dumped than break another's heart.

Broken heart is a brave heart,
Cautious heart is a coward heart.
Be stabbed in the back, no big deal,
But never be the cause of another's hurt.

12. Lunar Cycle (Sonnet 1432 - 1434)

Life's A Lunar Cycle
(The Sonnet, 1432)

Life is like the lunar cycle,
sometimes it is full shining,
sometimes it is half shining,
other times it goes totally dark.

But one thing is certain,
no one phase lasts forever,
it all just keeps changing,
thus light is sustained
through life's brief encounter.

The unpredictability of life
is what makes life predictable.
Sometimes it rains cats and dogs,
the next moment sunshine is unavoidable.

Sonnet 1433

No such thing as an uncreative heart,
If you are alive, you are creative.
Unless cluttered by status quo,
Every heart is by nature creative.

Heart alive is heart creative,
Creativity is a sign of life.
Uncreativity is pulselessness,
Symptom of a heart anemic of life.

I am not creative, I'm just alive,
Creativity is just a byproduct.
If you don't impose limits of norm,
Every blood vessel is creation-duct.

Plenticultural
(Sonnet 1434)

When I get mad, I revert to English,
because English is my first language.
When I feel romantic, I revert to Turkish,
because Turkish is my love language.

When I feel passionate, I revert to Spanish,
because Spanish is my passion language.
When I feel electric, I revert to Telugu,
because Telugu is my power language.

When nothing works, I revert to Korean,
because Korean is my backup language.
And you wonder why I never run empty,
why the natural spring is ever abundant!

Language is the gateway to culture,
Culture is the gateway to life.
I am no person who speaks many tongues,
I am the proof of plenticultural life.

13. Live (Sonnet 1435 - 1437)

Sonnet 1435

Human life by nature is plenticultural,
It's animal tradition that puts forth barrier.
Once the human truly musters their humanness,
All dividing tradition shall naturally wither.

Tradition divides, tradition unites;
Choose carefully the tradition you live.
Not all traditions imposed on you are good,
You gotta use conscience to pick and mix.

However, second-hand conscience won't do,
that you inherit from your ancestors.
If you can't muster conscience all on your own,
all conscience is without consequence.

Human life by nature is plenticultural,
which only feels blasphemy,
till you're one with the world.

Sonnet 1436

Human life is precious,
Don't clutter it with lies.
If you really wanna live,
Live original as life's ally.

Loyal to none for the sake of loyalty,
Obedient to none for the sake of obedience.
If you have an ounce of real human dignity,
Cast off obedience as living sapiens!

Life is too precious,
Don't vilify it with fear.
Most fears are second-hand fear,
Cast off identity of primitive heir.

Live, live and live again!
Live like you mean to live.
Past all ancestral forbiddance,
Live as lion, not infected sheep.

You Still Live
(Overcoming Grief Sonnet, 1437)

After your month long battle for breath,
Today I place you in nature's lap.
I know she'll care for you well,
like she once brought you to the world.

Fact of the matter is, you still live,
just in different form among the elements.
Nature's forces make us awake and restless,
Nature's forces coerce us into eternal rest.

There is no heaven, there is no hell,
these are concepts made by cowards.
Life is too sacred to be confined
by obsolete lies and superstitions.

Your light of affection shall continue
to shine bright in my memories.
You who was, nay, is like my second mother,
I won't say goodbye, for you still live.

14. Brainy (Sonnet 1438 - 1440)

Sonnet 1438

Life begins when I begin,
I begin when love begins.
Love begins when bond begins,
Bond begins past brainy leans.

Brain's got a role, sure enough,
not as driver, but as helper.
Heart's gotta decide whether to
take charge or let brain be the driver.

But we gotta be clear about one thing,
What does the term heart really mean?
The heart I speak of is
not merely a jumble of impulses,
but a symphony of sentiment and sentience.

Heart in practice isn't devoid of brain,
Heart in practice contains the brain.
The heart and brain divide is sheer fiction;
In everyday life, heart and brain act as one.

Sonnet 1439

Hearty and brainy conquers the world,
One can't be compromised for the other.
A dying world can be brought to life,
only when heart and truth act together.

Heart alive knows the worth of brain,
Hence, it never undermines reason.
Sometimes reason must take a backseat,
that doesn't make it redundant.

Only thing worth redundancy is apathy,
There is no place of arrogant coldness.
Cowards may use reason to justify apathy,
Here reason is not at fault, but the savages.

Life is too grand to discard
any of the potent mental faculties.
Foster awareness and you shall know,
which circumstances require which faculties.

Sonnet 1440

Ben senin kan kardeş olmayabilirim ama,
son nefesime kadar senin can kardeşinim.
Mutlu günlerinde beni bulamayabilirsin,
ama zor zamanlarda beni daima bulacaksın.

I may not be your blood brother,
In me you have a heart brother.
I may disappear in your happy days,
In difficult times I'll surely appear.

Difficulty shared is difficulty halved,
Happiness shared is happiness doubled.
Sickness acknowledged is half treated,
Wellness aware is wellness doubled.

Awareness is the highway to meaning and sapience.
Selflessness is the key to collective wholeness.

15. Family (Sonnet 1441 - 1443)

Bereavement Sermon
(The Sonnet, 1441)

You don't find a way out of grief,
You embrace it and it becomes your strength.
You don't find a way out of suffering,
You surf it and it endows you with courage.

Avoiding sorrow you won't find happiness,
Road to happiness goes through sorrow.
No matter how dark life seems tonight,
without heartwrecking darkness, we'll
never discover resilience, and grow.

Amidst the grief none of this makes sense,
I've felt it first hand this past month.
So I say, it's okay to be shattered to pieces,
but you must gather the pieces and soldier on,
for the sake of your living loved ones.

It's okay to not be okay, it means
your mind is trying to heal itself.
Persevering pain for those who live,
the sun will rise once again.

Sonnet 1442

Sooner or later the rain stops,
and the sun rises again.
Sooner or later the drought passes,
and greenery flourishes again.

Sooner or later tears turn treasure
and smile dawns again.
Sooner or later despair subsides,
and hope triumphs again.

Sooner or later the fog fades
and the path is revealed again.
Sooner or later the freeze thaws
and warmth seeps through again.

Sooner or later agony is tamed
and felicity is sighted again.
Sooner or later ominosity crumbles
and the glint of gaiety roars again.

Sonnet 1443

In this world nothing is permanent,
So don't chase after permanence.
Instead, cherish the impermanence,
and live each second doubly sentient.

Never miss a day to act your love,
for tomorrow may never come.
I say this with a boulder on my chest,
life exists today, not tomorrow.

So, shine my friend, shine bright
for those who mean to you the world.
In this moment, I say, be selfish,
let nothing compromise family love.

I'm a reformer, I chose the world over family,
but even I had to put the reformer aside
when tragedy struck my home.
As a commoner, you do as much as you can
for the world, but never let idealism
undermine the welfare of your home.

16. Gospel (Sonnet 1444 - 1446)

Sonnet 1444

Burn my friend, burn,
Burn so bright that
the sun gets fried!
Shine my friend, shine,
Shine so bright that
Rudolf goes blind!

Smile my friend, smile,
Smile so pure that
flowers shy away.
Love my friend, love,
Love so drunk that
Rumi himself lays the way.

Fly my friend, fly,
Fly so fearless that
Tagore himself honors you.
Live my friend, live,
Live so unchained that
time makes gospel of you.

Sonnet 1445

You are the gospel you need to read,
You are the path you need to walk.
You are the torch you need to light,
You are the voice you need to talk.

You are the sight you need to see,
You are the thirst you need to quench.
You are the warmth you need to wear,
You are the drought you need to drench.

You are the muck you need to mend,
You are the wrong you need to right.
You are the storm you need to brave,
You are the fate you need to write.

Sonnet 1446

I write poetry because
science tastes better as poetry.
I write poetry because
divinity tastes better as poetry.

I write poetry because
philosophy comes to life through poetry.
I write poetry because
sociology comes to life through poetry.

I write poetry because
theology gains humanity through poetry.
I write poetry because
legality gains humanity through poetry.

Then again, I don't write poetry,
It's poetry that writes me.
Amidst cold logic and blind faith,
poetry is reminder of humanity.

17. Dumb (Sonnet 1447 - 1449)

Sonnet 1447

Humans are so dumb that
even while speaking of emotion,
they can't help intellectualizing it.
Thus they invent nonsense
like emotional intelligence.

Humans are so dumb that
while speaking of knowledge,
they can't help quantifying it.
Thus they invent nonsense
like intelligence quotient.

Humans are so dumb that
even while speaking of divinity,
they can't help indoctrinating it.
Thus they invent nonsense
like scripture-based godliness.

AI Aftermath
(Sonnet 1448)

Today you pay for services of AI,
Tomorrow you'll pay for AI-free service.
Today you pay machines to replace humans,
Tomorrow you'll pay humans to overcome machines.

So no, I'm not worried that AI will replace humans,
Once the AI bubble bursts, humans will be priceless.
Sure, manual labor will be automated for good,
But human originality will be worth a king's ransom.

We shall move from labor-based job market
to creativity-based job market.
Once the honeymoon is over
humanity will come to its senses.

Today they pay machines
to make humans redundant,
Tomorrow they'll pay humans a fortune
to prevent humanity from going redundant.

Sonnet 1449

No species have caused
their own downfall,
unlike humans who are causing
their own extinction.

Worst kind of extinction is the one
caused in the name of progress.
Worst kind of downfall is the one
that comes in the shape of advancement.

That's why I say,
Be cautious of your ignorance,
but more cautious of your intelligence.
An intelligent species don't fall
due to lack of intelligence,
but due to arrogance of intelligence.

18. Immense (Sonnet 1450 - 1452)

Sonnet 1450

I have but one rule of reputation,
I never let Naskar open his mouth
except on keyboard and on stage,
all other times I am just regular Abi,

who is insecure like everybody else,
vulnerable like everybody else,
who is naive like everybody else,
easily fooled like everybody else.

Naturally it's easy to tread over Abi,
indeed most times he ends up the prey.
But every crisis that Abi encounters,
only adds to Naskar's immenseness.

Sonnet 1451

Naskar is immense
because Abi is humble.
Naskar is well aware
because Abi is stupid.

Naskar is fearless
because Abi is insecure.
Naskar is resolute
because Abi is clumsy.

Naskar is invincible
because Abi is vulnerable.
Naskar is incorruptible
because Abi is gullible.

Naskar is immortal
because Abi is mortal.
Naskar is impossible
because Abi is normal.

Sonnet 1452

We make ourselves immense,
We make ourselves narrow.
We choose whether we're whole,
or just more savages shallow.

Shallow or whole, it's up to us.
Kind or cruel, it's up to us.
Hardwired or heartwired, it's up to us.
Blunderlust or wonderlust, it's up to us.

Upon human choice unfolds cosmic destiny,
for the cosmos reflects in the mirror of mind.
As we dare, so we share -
the present of mindful lift
or the future of mindless night.

19. Spark (Sonnet 1453 - 1455)

Sonnet 1453

Narrowness from ancestors,
Immenseness from nature -
We gotta choose what's important,
Civil dawn or stoneage disaster.

Inheritance warrants scrutiny, not respect,
for not all inheritance is civilized.
If you can't tell good inheritance from bad,
no miracle can end your bouts of fright.

Humankind's most inherited
tendency has been intolerance -
till this changes nothing will change.
Till our supreme inheritance is integration,
all inheritance is decadence.

No inheritance is worth more than humanness,
No ancestry is worth more than humanity.
If your ancestors hand you over division,
Disown such ancestors, not your humanity.

Sonnet 1454

Our ancestors are secondary,
Our traditions are secondary,
Our religion is secondary,
Our culture is secondary,

Our scripture is secondary,
Our constitution is secondary,
Our nationality is secondary,
Our ethnicity is secondary,

Our rituals are secondary,
Our beliefs are secondary,
Our facts are secondary,
Our intelligence is secondary,

All else is secondary, save community.
All tribe is savage, save humanity.

Sonnet 1455

If you can't find God in
people, your God is dead.
If you can't find holiness in
people, your holiness is fake.

If you can't find life outside
the church, your church is dead.
If you can't find light beyond
the altar, your light is fake.

If you can't find truth outside your
scripture, your scripture is a lie.
If you can't find divinity outside
Vatican, your Vatican is a lie.

Divinity is uncanonable,
Churches and temples are obstacle.
If you can't find the holy spark
among the living, such is but
holiness of the jungle.

20. Inconvenient (Sonnet 1456 - 1458)

Sonnet 1456

The Islamic culture has made me a better poet,
The Western culture has made me a better scientist.
The Sanatana culture has made me a better philosopher,
The entire world has contributed to my wholeness.

Hence I am dutybound to empower
the good from every corner,
just as I am dutybound to call out
the inhumanities of every corner.

I admit, in the beginning I did
look upon America bit favorably.
But as the giant unfolded with truth,
gratitude no longer warranted partiality.

Today I can be grateful to a culture,
without being blind to its atrocities.
Even if it makes me inconvenient to many,
I prefer controversy over complicity.

Sonnet 1457

Look at the giant's present,
You'll witness triumph.
Look at the giant's past,
You'll discovery tragedy.

Look at the giant's successes,
You'll understand their capacity.
Look at the giant's failures,
You'll understand tenacity.

Giants are not giants
because of their victories,
giants are giants because of the
defeats to which they didn't submit.

There is no glory without agony,
no tenacity without treachery.
No transformation without turmoil,
there is no giant without tragedy.

Sonnet 1458

Wisdom unfolds when we're at our lowest,
Fog thickens when we're at our highest.
Be cautious of your shining victories,
Behind every victory lurks potential descent.

Triumph is more blinding than tragedy,
Applause is more blinding than mockery.
Look at USA to get a sense of this -
Madness of triumph made America
the United States of Atrocity.

Walk carefully in failure,
but more carefully in success.
One false move, and before you know,
you're a septic tank of derangement.

21. Idea (Sonnet 1459 - 1461)

The UAE Sonnet, 1459

I'm asked to compare USA with UAE,
So here it is, in my free form sonnetary.

For starters, there is no comparison -
UAE is a civilized country, USA is not.
Sure UAE has its share of violations,
like every living country in the world,

but unlike USA, the incredible growth
and the very birth of UAE is not founded
on the worst kind of atrocities in history.

In fact, forget the rich, safe and
prosperous UAE - on the civilization scale
USA is the bottom scraper of history.

Note: It took a lot of heartache to state without a doubt, that USA is not a civilized country. However, you must note that this entire statement is founded on the historic atrocities of America and the rising tendency of intolerance in the American society. Fact of the matter is, if you are white, straight and christian, America may be safe haven for you, but for everybody else, that's not the case.

Sonnet 1460

Every great idea is
unpopular in the beginning,
Every great idea is
unprofitable in the beginning.

But any idea founded on inhumanity,
is the antithesis of a great idea.
No matter how much you sugarcoat it,
poison cannot be treated as humanitarian.

All ideas must be scrutinized by conscience,
not by its outward shine and glory.
If it fails to provide collective lift,
it belongs in the trash, not on driver's seat.

A popular idea is not necessarily humane idea,
An economical idea isn't necessarily humane idea.
Mount Rushmore may be peddled as a historic site,
At the end of the day, it is criminal americana.

Sonnet 1461

A popular idea isn't
necessarily a worthwhile idea.
Take Marvel for example -
a name that was once synonymous
with cinematic splendor.

The only reason Marvel matters today
is due to its representation factor -
other than that, Marvel lost its
cinematic magic long time ago,
right after the first Avengers movie.

As a matter of fact,
the first Avengers movie
was the last Avengers movie.
It's easy to be creative for a short while,
but to sustain creativity over time
is an act of real genius.

That's why, though most may not notice it,
but I've slowed down from my usual pace,
because I've already achieved
all the landmarks I wanted to achieve.

22. Fall (Sonnet 1462 - 1464)

Sonnet 1462

Better slow down than bog down!
Better take a breather than asphyxiate.
I repeat, better modulate your pace wisely,
than boneheadedly rush to derangement.

Clean head requires occasional breaks,
It's not a break if it replenishes.
If you say you need no replenishment,
you're the herald of your own downfall.

I admit, even I used to feel an insane rush,
till I finished my centurion sermon.
Once I crossed my landmark hundred,
an inexplicable calm took over my mind.

Now there is no rush, no hurry -
I've given the world ample thunder
to last for generations to come.
Everything I write now is sheer bonus,
with no strict deadline for publication.

Sonnet 1463

When you write, cherish the writing.
When you code, cherish the coding.
When you sing, cherish the singing.
When you love, cherish loving.

Whatever you do, do it with love -
without the rush to reach a conclusion.
Life is a journey from question to question,
there is no such thing as an ultimate solution.

Live life like there's no other way,
Fall in love like nothing else matters.
Cast cowardice and insecurity into the ocean,
Swim through tsunami like the sea is your empire.

Contract Matrimony
(The Sonnet, 1464)

When I fall, I fall wholly -
without a safety net of any kind.
Prenups are an insult of love,
all in fear of an imaginary night.

Contract lovers are worse
than contract killers,
at least contract killers
don't second guess their motive.
Either love or don't,
there's no second guessing -
either marry or don't,
there's no contract matrimony.

Prenups are for juveniles,
Clauses are for cowards.
To seek escape in commitment,
is an act of con, not love.

Escapists have no right to love,
Lovers have no need for escape.
When you change exes like socks,
It's a sickness, not a choice.

23. Asset (Sonnet 1465 - 1467)

Honor and Love
(The Sonnet, 1465)

I don't care for one time fling,
Got no hankering for casual coitus.
I am a human, not baboon set free,
I don't consent to rampant desires.

When I fall I fall mind and body,
Body plays a little, more the mind.
I'm attracted to face, not figure,
Finally by mind the deal is signed.

If the mind doesn't come through,
a cute face doesn't sustain nothing.
Heart anemic makes the world anemic,
getting drunkly sick on perverted fling.

In a world of cheats and perves,
Be the proof of honor and love.
In the wild of sharks and wolves,
Be the gentle elephant, be a dove.

Sonnet 1466

I am conscience,
I am honor.
I am commitment,
I am character.

My greatest asset is not my legacy,
My greatest asset is my character.
It's character that legitimizes legacy,
Without which, all legacy is dishonor.

Legacy without honor is garbage,
Honor is the supreme legacy.
Lose legacy, lost something.
Lose honor, lost everything.

I am conscience,
backed by honor.
I am commitment,
powered by character.

Sonnet 1467

Character, my identity;
Conscience, my guide.
Honor is my defense,
Heart is my tide.

Simplicity, my lifestyle;
Awareness, my way.
Accountability, my principle,
from which I'll never sway.

I don't have a publisher behind me,
I don't have an institution behind me,
I don't have an industry behind me,
I only have my mission of undivided humanity.

My mission is my reason,
My mission is my cause.
I work to live my mission,
not for a bucketful applause.

24. Turmoil (Sonnet 1468 - 1470)

Sonnet 1468

Every time right around
the 70th sonnet I run empty.
So I pick up from the emptiness,
And lo, I regain continuity.

This is how life works,
sometimes empty, sometimes whole.
Embrace the moment in its fullness,
thus rises momentum, lo and behold!

You can't fight the tide,
You either surf or sink.
You can't fight time,
You either dare or drown.

Time is forged from the fabric of uncertainty,
only the brave can turn it in favor of a purpose.
The more you resist the turmoil of time,
more you're reminded of your insignificance.

Sonnet 1469

From the fabric of
uncertainty time is forged.
This very fabric is
all the arsenal we've got.

Only the brave can
carve it at will,
while the cowards cower
behind the excuse of fate.

Those who got no backbone,
talk of fate and destiny,
while the sapiens with spine,
is up and about doing their duty.

No change comes about through sheeply civilians,
Lionheart leaders are needed in every corner.
Lions don't leave society in the hands of government.
Government is second in command -
civilians, chief commander.

Dear li'l governments
(The Sonnet, 1470)

Dear li'l governments of the world,

You don't have a friend in me,
If people are not your priority.
You don't have a friend in me,
If you thrive on inequality.

You don't have a friend in me,
If you're partial to one religion.
You don't have a friend in me,
If you're founded on nationalism.

Dear li'l governments of the world,
If you know what's best for you,
Walk the course of integration.
If you choose tribalism instead,
In me you'll find your abolition.

25. Answer (Sonnet 1471 - 1473)

156

Sonnet 1471

There is no law but the human,
There is no bible but the human.
There is no koran but the human,
There is no cosmos but the human.

There is no ghost but the human,
There is no god but the human.
There is no art but the human,
There is no science but the human.

There is no reason but the human,
There is no faith but the human.
There is no cause but the human,
There is no effect but the human.

There is no question but the human,
There is no answer but the human.
While apes are busy chasing myths,
Humans emerge as illumination.

Everybody is a terrorist,
till you see the reformist
(The Sonnet, 1472)

Everybody is a president,
till you see the first servant.
Everybody is king kong,
till emerges the first sapiens.

Everybody is marconi,
till you meet the Nikola.
Everybody is prime minister,
till you see the transformer.

Everybody is mercenary,
till you see the tsunami.
Everybody is a godman,
till awakens commoner godly.

Everybody is police,
till comes the vessel of peace.
Everybody is a terrorist,
till you see the reformist.

Sonnet 1473

No ideology but reform,
my identity is reformer.
No fundamental but union,
my duty is of unifier.

I am a sufi - a sufi believes
in love* and kindness.
I am an advaitin -
an advaitin believes
in universal oneness.

Bodhisattva to Buddha,
I'm the spirit of humanistana.
I am the fabled Yehova -
the state of unbarred *ahava.

I am all, I am the one.
I am the father, I am the son.

26. Promise (Sonnet 1474 - 1476)

Sonnet 1474

I am all, I am the one.
I am the father, I am the son.

I am the divine,
I am the common.
I am life's code,
I am the python.

(Rumi-ka bhai,
Shakespeare-ka baap.
Naam hai Visvavictor,
Manavta-ka jawaab!

Hermano de Rumi,
Padre de Shakespeare.
Nombre Visvavictor,
Servir es vivir!

Mevlana'nin kardeşi,
Bard'ın babası.
Adım Vicdansaadet,
Halkın koruması!)

Brother of Rumi,
Father of the Bard.
Name is Visvavictor,
Humankind's vangaurd!

I am the father, I am the son.
I am the mecca, I am evolution.

Sonnet 1475

Vadi in turkish means valley,
Vaada in hindi means promise.
In the valley of promise I'm dervish,
whom you can't fathom without oneness.

I am the promise of love over law,
I am the promise of undoctrination.
I am the promise of heart over hate,
I'm the denouncing of customary division.

I am the act of conscience over custom,
I am the defender of breath of the living.
I am the keeper of love in the cosmos,
I'm the divine bulldozer of hatebusting.

To hell with tradition, to hell with custom!
To hell with slavery sold as vision!

Sonnet 1476

In a world of trolls and perves,
Be the ray of truth and love.
In the wild of sharks and wolves,
Be the gentle elephant, be a dove.

(If you got nothing good to say,
don't say nothing at all.
Unless they are a threat
to society like the 2017 Potus,
don't diss a person for their
little shortfalls.)

Boasting through bigotry,
while bigots mock the lover,
stand true to your core of love,
never dwindle in the face of sneer.

Never try to hide your wounds,
Wear your wounds as divine ornament.
Human wounds are the source of wonder,
Wounds wielded are ointment manifested.

The difference between wound
and ointment is in attitude.
In a world that exploits wounds,
be humanity's ointment resolute.

27. Smile (Sonnet 1477 - 1479)

Sonnet 1477

I am out of ointment
so I let my wounds bleed.
Lo, the dusk turns to morn,
bearing the gift of glee!

Blank slate is a divine call,
a call to paint the divine valley,
a valley where life is one with life,
made of living love, not fantasy.

Oye monsoon, come -
Wash my tears away!
Can't hold back any longer,
now the storm must break!

Here, I give in -
let the tears break!
I refuse pain no more,
I persevere smiling awake!

Sonnet 1478

Smiling through martyrdom,
I magnetize magnanimity.
One sacrifice awakens millions,
One life resuscitates humanity.

Only the selfless can
die a million times
and still keep on living.
Only the heart can shatter
to a million pieces
and still keep beating,

Injury to ointment,
heartbreak to daybreak -
ordeal for the tourist,
calling for the traveler.

Fret not the torment,
torment builds tenacity.
Cherish the whole climb,
Climb makes the character.

Sonnet 1479

If you haven't felt like
giving up at times,
you haven't struggled enough.
If you haven't bounced back
from occasional doubts,
your conviction hasn't toughened enough.

If you haven't pondered
the futility of life,
you haven't lived enough.
If you haven't conquered
the futility of life,
you haven't grown enough.

If you haven't developed an ear
to listen past the unspoken,
you haven't developed hearing.
If you haven't developed an eye
to look past the obvious,
you haven't developed a sight.

28. Imprints (Sonnet 1480 - 1482)

174

Sonnet 1480

If you can't say anything but
my religion says this,
my religion says that,
I got no interest in hearing you.

If you can't say anything but
science says this,
science says that,
I got no interest in hearing you.

If you can't say anything but
philosophy says this,
philosophy says that,
I got no interest in hearing you.

If you can't say anything but
psychology says this,
psychology says that,
I got no interest in hearing you.

If you can't utter a single word
without parroting second-hand thought,
my phone deserves more attention than you.
But grow up and muster one original idea,
I'll put aside my writing to listen to you.

Sonnet 1481

Think one thing,
but think it original,
if not, you ain't a living being,
just a dead loudmouth fossil.

If you wanna think, think alive.
If you wanna live, live human.
Fossils look good in the museum,
They have no role in civilization.

Sure, I shall fade too, but
not for a few thousand years yet.
I decide the parameters of my demise,
I am no pawn to time's cosmic chess.

I am the emperor of time and space,
I am the backbone of human universe.
With my hands I carve civilization,
I am awareness absolute - I am sapiocosmos.

From Ape to Human
(The Sonnet, 1482)

To label a spirit is to cripple a spirit,
What we call cultural imprints are prison.
Society of such culture is no human society,
but merely an overglorified animal kingdom.

Sure, the culture we're born in are part of us,
But it must never take over human identity.
That's how heritage facilitates bias-n-hate,
And culture becomes excuse for inhumanity.

Call it advaita, nirvana or humanity,
the purpose is to surpass all divide.
Anything that distances mind from mind,
must never be defended as cultural pride.

Mission is, not to remove cultural imprints,
But to be civilized enough to surpass them.
Only then can we be the bridge of benevolence,
Only then the glorified ape shall emerge as human.

29. Alley (Sonnet 1483 - 1485)

Sonnet 1483

I am not interested in intellectual discourse,
I am not interested in religious discourse.
Close your eyes, turn off facts and fiction;
There's an alley leading from my heart to yours.

I roam the valley unattained by metaphysics,
I'm the pedestrian of light beyond logic.
I don't deny the need for logic or fantasy,
But why blemish bonding by freezing logic!

Sure, there are people who bond over logic,
Like there are people who bond over fiction.
I am not content with the narrowness of either,
For there's more to life than facts and fiction.

Close your eyes, put aside faith and intellect;
There's an alley leading from my heart to yours.
Facts and fiction all have their time and place,
But first, come, let's walk the human shores!

Sonnet 1484

More than being the spark of reason,
Be the reason for someone's spark.
Better than bearing the light of faith,
Instill faith in someone's light.

The faith I speak of is faith of life,
not the faith of dogmas and doctrines.
Amidst all fancy candles in darkness,
Be the one human candle in coldness.

Intellect don't impress me much,
Devoutness of doctrine repulses me.
Have you ever made a stranger smile,
Ever left your seat to the elderly!

Sonnet 1485

Passing clouds I meet plenty,
But beautiful persistence I meet few.
That's why I care what they feel,
Even though I pretend it's all cool.

I got used to hearing racial slurs,
So they bother me no longer.
But when a kind heart disappears,
It does leave me to wonder.

Naskar is beyond opinion,
His conviction invincible;
Abi is just a regular person,
He is trusting, hence vulnerable.

The invincibility of Naskar comes
from the vulnerability of Abi.
To the world I may be shaktimaan,
In everyday life, I'm gangadhar shastry.

30. Vulnerable (Sonnet 1486 - 1488)

Sonnet 1486

To be vulnerable is to be human,
But not at the expense of your honor.
In love there is no honor and dishonor,
Not everyone is worth ruining your honor.

If someone is interested,
they'll find time -
If not, they'll find excuse.
You can only reach out,
rest is not up to you.

Let them be as they please,
Keep your honor, after you've tried.
Don't ruin your honor for no reason,
Loss of honor is worse than loss of life.

Sonnet 1487

Life is honor, honor is life,
Only thing higher is love.
In love you may risk it all,
In any other circumstance,
compromise honor, you must not.

Honor and honesty go together;
No honesty, no honor.
Cowards lie, liars cower;
Truth is the greatest reliever.

Every lie is a burden,
that takes a toll on life.
Unless a truth is actually inhuman,
never succumb to the lure of lie.

Sonnet 1488

Every lie is a burden,
that takes a toll on life.
Unless the truth is inhuman,
never succumb to the lure of lie.

How can truth be inhuman -
if you ask this,
you're yet to experience life.
Truth is not always humane,
in which case, you gotta
let your heart decide.

Prioritize life, not truth;
Let truth serve life,
not the other way around.
Modulate honesty adapting to life,
Do what does good to the world around.

31. Fancy (Sonnet 1489 - 1491)

Sonnet 1489

I'll be honest with you,
I know nothing about writing poetry.
All my sonnets you're crazy about,
they wrote themselves through me.

Every time I try to write, it's drab;
only when the sonnets write me it's fab.
So I gave up writing anything from thought,
the heart takes over, and lo pours divine swag.

No need to mystify this with superstition,
It just means I'm not in control of my magic.
Perhaps that's why I'm born in the first place,
to be the fountainhead of miracle release.

Hence, I learnt to trust the miracle,
I never force my words on paper.
I wait patient for monsoon to come,
and sure enough, the drought disappears.

Sonnet 1490

Aim for exponential productivity,
life will pass you by without knowing.
Be productive, sure, but within balance,
otherwise, it is all degrading.

Aim for exponential progress,
and sooner or later you'll regret it.
It's expansion that brings contentment,
It's expansion that brings balance.

Expansion is an act of mindfulness,
Exponential progress is an act of mindlessness.
Such progress only ruins the sweetness of life,
Leaving behind a pompous wreck of fancy citadels.

Progress is no progress if it
ruins the soul of humanity.
If you forget what it's to be human,
such progress is crime against humanity.

Sonnet 1491

Don't confuse progress with uplift,
Don't confuse contacts with connection.
Don't confuse convenience with advancement,
Don't confuse machine learning with education.

From the tiniest speck of neuron
to an entire sapient person,
we always look for connection.
If you say, you don't need connection,
it doesn't mean you're strong,
it means you are dead and rotten.

Exponential progress is catalyst of coldness,
all peddled in the name of advancement.
Monkeys burn millions selling you the future,
while back on earth humans struggle to make
ends meet on 1/4 to 7 dollar hourly wage.

32. Living (Sonnet 1492 - 1494)

Sonnet 1492

If you cared more about
making people smile
than bringing machines to life,
we'd be at a much better place.

With all the tech we have today,
we could equalize the world tomorrow.
But no, cyborgs gotta develop more,
they feel impotent unless their tentacles grow.

That's why, neither genocide nor invasion
must obstruct the growth of apely machines.
It's okay if children die of malnourishment,
funding mustn't cease for glorious tech fiends.

Terrestrial terrains to celestial shores,
humanity is the only species to die of smart-ness.
If we cared more about people than devices,
truly and honestly, we'd be at a much better place.

Sonnet 1493

Awake, arise, o heartforce of earth,
Get down to the gutter of society!
Clean up the mess left by cleverclogs,
Put them in place instilling sanity.

When cyborgs try to undermine humanity,
Take charge and stand as their guardian.
When bigots try to raise walls of hate,
Walk as messiah and be their salvation.

Bigots and cyborgs are the enemies of life,
Treat them as your children gone wrong.
Hate not, harm them not, for they're sick;
Buy them flowers and help their rehabilitation.

Sonnet 1494

Connect with folks,
more than your phone.
Connect with life,
more than wifi.

Foster meaningful connection,
not mindless contacts.
Nourish your life wide awake,
not package it in old rags.

Abandon the rags you call heritage,
Learn to look with living eyes.
Be a zealous mind, not a xerox machine,
why do you chain yourself to lies!

Be the lifeforce of the present,
and all good things shall follow.
Monkeys may chase after past and future,
You be human and prioritize the moment.

33. Vision (Sonnet 1495 - 1497)

Sonnet 1495

We've got to spare some attention
in studying the past and
contemplating the future, but never
at the expense of the present.

Note that I use the words
studying and contemplating,
which are not the same as
conforming and obsessing.

Study the past to
learn from mistakes,
Contemplate the future
to build the present.

We can never really build the future,
We can only build the present.
To chase the future abandoning the present,
isn't an act of vision, but derangement.

Sonnet 1496

True vision enhances our human sight,
It doesn't blind us with obsession.
True vision delivers us from fright,
It doesn't add to our castration.

True vision helps us overcome bias,
It doesn't envelop us with new bias.
True vision helps us conquer the lies,
It doesn't peddle us sophisticated lies.

True vision emboldens our human spine,
not replace it with artificial slime.
True vision brings down all the barriers,
not create walls of a different kind.

True vision enhances us as human beings,
it doesn't separate us from ourselves.
True vision adds to the meaning of life,
it doesn't add to the narrowness of apes.

Sonnet 1497

I often reach out to strangers,
who seem aligned with my heart.
To hell with unspoken laws of fame,
I wanna know each of you by heart!

I care nothing about maintaining distance,
I wanna sit with each of you and talk.
Often this naivety gets me into trouble,
often the fans turn out to be trolls-n-perves.

Still I learn nothing from the bad encounters,
I still crave reaching out to each and every one.
My heart isn't fashioned to favor distance,
I live, breathe and die of assimilation.

I got no regrets for the times I'm exploited,
It's the rough and tumble of a reformer's life.
Amidst the sea of dampened destitution,
I am just a spark of untamed light.

34. Present (Sonnet 1498 – 1500)

Sonnet 1498

Advancement doesn't mean walking with blinkers,
Enlightenment is the antithesis of condescension.
If your vision doesn't bring you closer to people,
You are a textbook case of moral destitution.

Feminism doesn't mean walking half-naked,
though it's alright, if that's what you choose.
Freedom doesn't mean drinking and smoking,
though it's alright, if that's what you choose.

Learn to get your priorities straight,
Put focus where focus is due.
If you just change the shape of insanity,
It's not revolution but devolution renewed.

Neither burqa nor bikini is the sign of progress,
they only depict personal choice, nothing more.
Grow out of clothes, and look into character,
only then you'll get to see the sapiens glow.

Sonnet 1499

Where clothes are trivial,
character is prime -
where machines are trivial,
mind is prime -

where religion is trivial,
reform is prime -
where wealth is trivial,
wonder is prime -

where alcohol is trivial,
aspiration, prime -
where middlefinger, trivial,
mindfulness is prime -

that, is the world I call human,
where one reflects all, all reflect one.

My Struggle
(Sonnet 1500)

My struggle is to build a world, where
gestapo, mi6, cia, raw, all are history;
where thieves aren't glorified as heroes,
invasion isn't sugarcoated as security;

military is found only in books of history,
where guns are displayed in museum as relics;
nukes are just defense against celestial threat,
where green sources power all things electric;

where it's illegal to amass limitless wealth -
food, housing, education, healthcare, are free;
where no one can be politician without license,
where citizens listen to experts, not celebrity.

My struggle is to build a world, where
human rights is a human issue, not legal one;
where equality is not a belief, but the norm -
where human is neither ape nor robot, but human.

BIBLIOGRAPHY

Archer M., (2000), Being Human: The Problem of Agency. Cambridge University Press.

Adolphs R (2003) Cognitive neuroscience of human social behaviour. Nature Rev Neurosci 4: 165–178.

Adolphs R, Tranel D, Damasio AR (2003) Dissociable neural systems for recognizing emotions. Brain Cogn 52: 61–69.

Andresen, Jensine, and Robert Forman, eds. Cognitive Models and Spiritual Maps. Bowling Green, Ohio: Imprint Academic, 2000.

Azari, Nina, Janpeter Nickel, Gilbert Wunderlich, Michael Niedeggen, Harald Hefter, Lutz Tellmann, Hans Herzog, Petra Stoerig, Dieter Birnbacher, and Rudiger Seitz. "Neural

Correlates of Religious Experience." European Journal of Neuroscience 13, no. 8 (2001)

Agar, N. (2004). Liberal eugenics: In defence of human enhancement. London: Blackwell Publishing.

Bernstein R.J., (1976), The Restructuring Social and Political Thought.

Bernstein R.J., (1983), Beyond Relativism and Objectivism: Science, Hermeneutics, and Praxis. Philadelphia: University of Pennsylvania Press.

Bernstein R.J., (1986), Philosophical Profiles. Philadelphia: University of Pennsylvania Press.

Birkhead, T. R., Johnson, S. D. & Nettleship, D. N. (1985). Extra-pair matings and mate guarding in the common murre Uria aalge. - Anim. Behav. 33, p. 608-619.

Beauregard, Mario, and Vincent Paquette. "Neural Correlates of a Mystical Experience in Carmelite Nuns." Neuroscience Letters 405, no. 3 (2006)

Benson, Herbert. Timeless Healing: The Power and Biology of Belief. New York: Scribner, 1996

Bose, Subhas Chandra. An Indian Pilgrim: An Unfinished Autobiography, Oxford University Press, 1997

Bogen, J.E.(1995a), 'On the neurophysiology of consciousness: Part I. An overview', Consciousness and Cognition, 4.

Bogen, J.E. (1995b), 'On the neurophysiology of consciousness: Part II. Constraining the semantic problem', Consciousness and Cognition, 4.

Bremner, J. D., R. Soufer, et al. (2001). "Gender differences in cognitive and neural correlates of remembrance of emotional words." Psychopharmacol Bull 35 (3).

Brothers, L. (2002). The social brain: A project for integrating primate behavior and neurophysiology in a new domain. In J. T. Cacioppo et al. (Eds.), Foundations in neuroscience. Cambridge, MA: MIT Press.

Buss, D. D. (2003). Evolutionary Psychology: The New Science of Mind, 2nd ed. New York: Allyn & Bacon.

Buss, D. M. (1989). "Conflict between the sexes: Strategic interference and the evocation of anger and upset." J Pers Soc Psychol 56 (5).

Buss, D. M. (1995). "Psychological sex differences. Origins through sexual selection." Am Psychol 50 (3).

Buss, D. M., and D. P. Schmitt (1993). "Sexual strategies theory: An evolutionary perspective on human mating." Psychol Rev 100 (2).

Blakemore SJ, Decety J (2001) From the perception of action to the understanding of intention. Nature Rev Neurosci 2: 561.

Carr L, Iacoboni M, Dubeau MC, Mazziotta JC, Lenzi GL (2003) Neural mechanisms of empathy in humans: a relay from neural systems for imitation to limbic areas. Proc Natl Acad Sci USA 100: 5497–5502.

Chomsky Noam, (2017) Requiem for the American Dream

Chomsky Noam, (2016) Who Rules the World?

Chomsky Noam, (2010) How the World Works

Churchland, P.S. (1986), Neurophilosophy (Cambridge, MA: The MIT Press).

Churchland, P.S. & Ramachandran, V.S. (1993), 'Filling in: Why Dennett is wrong', in Dennett and His Critics:

Demystifying Mind, ed. B. Dahlbom (Oxford: Blackwell Scientific Press).

Churchland, P.S., Ramachandran, V.S. & Sejnowski, T.J. (1994), 'A critique of pure vision', in Large- scale Neuronal Theories of the Brain, ed. C. Koch & J.L. Davis (Cambridge, MA: The MIT Press).

Coyle EF. Integration of the physiological factors determining endurance performance ability. Exerc Sport Sci Rev. 1995;23:25–63.

Crick, F. (1994), The Astonishing Hypothesis: The Scientific Search for the Soul (New York: Simon and Schuster).

Crick, F. (1996), 'Visual perception: rivalry and consciousness', Nature, 379.

Crick, F. & Koch, C. (1992), 'The problem of consciousness', Scientific American, 267.

Damasio, A (2003a) Looking for Spinoza. Harcourt Inc. Damasio A (2003b) Feeling of emotion and the self. Ann NY Acad Sci 1001: 253–261.

d'Aquili, Eugene. "Senses of Reality in Science and Religion." Zygon 17, no 4 (1982)

d'Aquili, Eugene. "The Biopsychological Determinants of Religious Ritual Behavior." Zygon 10, no. 1 (1975)

Daly DD. 1958. Ictal affect. Am J Psychiatry.

Damasio, A. (1999) The Feeling of What Happens: Body, Emotion and the Making of Consciousness. London, Heinemann.

Darwin, C. (1859) On the Origin of Species by Means of Natural Selection. London, Murray.

Darwin, C. (1871) The Descent of Man and Selection in Relation to Sex. London, John Murray.

Darwin, C. (1872) The Expression of the Emotions in Man and Animals. London, John Murray; also published 1965, Chicago, University of Chicago Press.

Dawkins, R. (1976) The Selfish Gene. Oxford, Oxford University Press; a new edition, with additional material, was published in 1989.

Dewhurst, Kenneth, and A. W. Beard. "Sudden Religious Conversions in Temporal Lobe Epilepsy." British Journal of Psychiatry 117 (1970)

Dewhurst K, Beard AW. Sudden religious conversions in temporal lobe epilepsy. 1970 Epilepsy Behav 2003

Devinsky O, Lai G. Spirituality and religion in epilepsy. Epilepsy Behav 2008.

Devinsky, O., Morrell, MJ, Vogt, BA. (1995) 'Contribution of anterior cingulate cortex to behavior', Brain, 118.

E. Horvitz, "One Hundred Year Study on Artificial Intelligence: Reflections and Framing," ed: Stanford University, 2014.

Eckhart Meister, Selected Writings

Farah, M.J. (1989), 'The neural basis of mental imagery', Trends in Neurosciences, 10.

Freud, S. "The Interpretation of Dreams", 1900

Freud, S. "Selected papers on hysteria and other psychoneuroses" Journal of Nervous and Mental Disease 1909.

Freud, S. "The Origin and Development of Psychoanalysis", 1910

Freud, S. "Psychopathology of everyday life", 1914

Freud, S. "Beyond the Pleasure Principle", 1920

Frith, C.D. & Dolan, R.J. (1997), 'Abnormal beliefs: Delusions and memory', Paper presented at the May, 1997, Harvard Conference on Memory and Belief.

Gray JA. The Psychology of Fear and Stress. 2nd ed. New York, NY: Cambridge University Press; 1988.

Gloor, P. (1992), 'Amygdala and temporal lobe epilepsy', in The Amygdala: Neurobiological Aspects of Emotion, Memory and Mental Dysfunction, ed J.P. Aggleton (New York: Wiley-Liss).

Grady, D. (1993), 'The vision thing: Mainly in the brain', Discover, June.

Gallese V, Keysers C, Rizzolatti G (2004) A unifying view of the basis of social cognition. Trends Cogn Sci 8: 396–403.

Guevara Che, The Motorcycle Diaries, 1992

Hari R, Forss N, Avikainen S, Kirveskari S, Salenius S, Rizzolatti G (1998) Activation of human primary motor cortex during action observation: a neuromagnetic study. Proc. Natl Acad Sci USA 95: 15061–15065.

Hardy, G. H. (1940). Ramanujan. Cambridge: Cambridge University Press.

Hall, Daniel, Keith Meador, and Harold Koenig. "Measuring Religiousness in Health Research: Review and Critique." Journal of Religion and Health 47, no. 2 (2008)

Harris, Sam, Jonas Kaplan, Ashley Curiel, Susan Bookheimer, Marco Iacoboni, and Mark Cohen. "The Neural Correlates of Religious and Nonreligious Belief." PLoS One 4, no. 10 (October 1, 2009)

Halgren, E. (1992), 'Emotional neurophysiology of the amygdala within the context of human cognition', in The Amygdala: Neurobiological Aspects of Emotion, Memory and Mental Dysfunction, ed J.P. Aggleton (New York: Wiley-Liss).

Handbook of Emotions, Edited by Michael Lewis, Jeannette M. Haviland-Jones, and Lisa Feldman Barrett, The Guilford Press; 3rd edition (2010).

Hameroff, S.R. and Penrose, R. (1996) Conscious events as orchestrated space-time selections. Journal of Consciousness Studies 3(1), 36-53; also reprinted in J. Shear (ed.) (1997) Explaining Consciousness-The Hard Problem. Cambridge, MA, MIT Press, 177-95.

Haugeland, J. (ed.) (1997) Mind Design II: Philosophy, Psychology, Artificial Intelligence. Cambridge, MA, MIT Press.

Hauser, M.D. (2000) Wild Minds: What Animals Really Think. New York, Henry Holt and Co.; London, Penguin.

Hebb, D.O. (1949) The Organization of Behavior. New York, Wiley.

Hess, EH (1975) "The role of pupil size in communication," Scientific American, 233(5), 110–12.

Heyes, C.M. (1998) Theory of mind in nonhuman primates. Behavioral and Brain Sciences 21, 101-48; with commentaries.

Heyes, C.M. and Galef, B.G. (eds) (1996) Social Learning in Animals: The Roots of Culture. San Diego, CA, Academic Press.

Hilgard, E.R. (1986) Divided Consciousness: Multiple Controls in Human Thought and Action. New York, Wiley.

Hilton, E.N., Lundberg, T.R. Transgender Women in the Female

Category of Sport: Perspectives on Testosterone Suppression and Performance Advantage. Sports Med 51, 199–214 (2021).

Hitler, Adolf. Mein Kampf, 1925

Holt, J. (1999) Blindsight in debates about qualia. Journal of Consciousness Studies 6(5), 54-71.

Holloway RL (1996) Evolution of the human brain. In: Lock A, Peters CR (eds) Handbook of human symbolic evolution. Oxford University Press, Oxford

Jackson, F. (1982) Epiphenomenal qualia. Philosophical Quarterly 32, 127-36.

James, W. (1890) The Principles of Psychology (2 volumes). London, Macmillan.

James, W. (1902) The Varieties of Religious Experience: A Study in

Human Nature. New York and London, Longmans, Green and Co.

Jay, M. (ed.) (1999) Artificial Paradises: A Drugs Reader. London, Penguin.

Jaynes, J. (1976) The Origin of Consciousness in the Breakdown of the Bicameral Mind. New York, Houghton Mifflin.

Johnson, M.K. and Raye, C.L. (1981) Reality monitoring. Psychological Review 88, 67-85.

Kadim I, Mahgoub O, Baqir S et al. (2015) Cultured meat from muscle stem cells: a review of challenges and prospects. J Integr Agr 14: 222–233

Kandel, E. R. In Search of Memory: The Emergence of a New Science of Mind, W. W. Norton & Company (2007).

Kandel E. R. Schwartz JH, Jessel TM. Principles of neural sciences. New York; McGraw Hill, 2000.

Kihlstrom, J.F. (1996) Perception without awareness of what is perceived, learning without awareness of what is learned. In M. Velmans (ed.) The Science of Consciousness. London, Routledge, 23-46.

Kjaer, Troels, Camilla Bertelsen, Paola Piccini, David Brooks, Jorgen Alving, and Hans Lou. "Increased Dopamine Tone during Meditation- Induced Change of Consciousness." Cognitive Brain Research 13, no. 2 (April 2002)

Kölmel HW. 1985. Complex visual hallucinations in the hemianopic field. J Neurol Neurosurg Psychiatry.

Koenig, Harold. "Research on Religion, Spirituality, and Mental Health: A Review." Canadian Journal of Psychiatry 54, no. 5 (May 2009)

Koenig, Harold, ed. Handbook of Religion and Mental Health. San Diego, CA: Academic Press, 1998

Kraepelin E. Psychiatry: A Textbook for Students and Physicians. New York, NY: Science History Publications; 1990.

Lauglin, Charles, John McManus, and Eugene d'Aquili. Brain, Symbol, and Experience. 2nd ed. New York: Columbia University Press, 1992

LeDoux, J. E. (1996). The emotional brain. New York: Simon & Schuster.

LeDoux, J.E. (1992), 'Emotion and the amygdala', in The Amygdala: Neurobiological Aspects of Emo- tion, Memory and Mental Dysfunction, ed J.P. Aggleton (New York: Wiley-Liss).

Levin, D.T. and Simons, D.J. (1997) Failure to detect changes to attended objects in motion pictures. Psychonomic Bulletin and Review 4, 501-6.

Levine,J. (1983) Materialism and qualia: the explanatory gap. Pacific Philosophical Quarterly 64, 354-61.

Lewicki, P., Czyzewska, M. and Hoffman, H. (1987) Unconscious acquisition of complex procedural knowledge. Journal of Experimental Psychology: Learning, Memory and Cognition 13, 523-30.

Lewicki, P., Hill, T. and Czyzewska, M. (1992) Nonconscious acquisition of information. American Psychologist 47, 796-801.

Naskar, Abhijit. "Homo: A Brief History of Consciousness", 2015

Naskar, Abhijit. "What is Mind?", 2016

Naskar, Abhijit. "Love, God & Neurons: Memoir of A Scientist who found himself by getting lost", 2016

Naskar, Abhijit. "Principia Humanitas", 2017

Naskar, Abhijit. "We Are All Black: A Treatise on Racism", 2017

Naskar, Abhijit. "Either Civilized or Phobic: A Treatise on Homosexuality", 2017

Naskar, Abhijit. "The Bengal Tigress: A Treatise on Gender Equality", 2017

Naskar, Abhijit. "Morality Absolute", 2017

Naskar, Abhijit. "Build Bridges not Walls: In the name of Americana", 2018

Naskar, Abhijit. "Fabric of Humanity", 2018

Naskar, Abhijit. "Citizens of Peace: Beyond the Savagery of Sovereignty", 2019

Naskar, Abhijit. "The Constitution of The United Peoples of Earth", 2019

Naskar, Abhijit. "Neurons Giveth, Neurons Taketh Away | Abhijit Naskar | TEDxIIMRanchi", 2019 https://www.youtube.com/watch?v=BNX-Q0ySm80

Naskar, Abhijit. "Mission Reality", 2019

Naskar, Abhijit. "Operation Justice: To Make A Society That Needs No Law", 2019

Naskar, Abhijit. "Every Generation Needs Caretakers: The Gospel of Patriotism", 2020

Naskar, Abhijit. "Hurricane Humans: Give me accountability, I'll give you peace", 2020

Naskar, Abhijit. "Revolution Indomable", 2020

Naskar, Abhijit. "Servitude is Sanctitude", 2020

Naskar, Abhijit. "Good Scientist: When Science and Service Combine", 2020

Newberg, Andrew. "How God Changes Your Brain: An Introduction to Jewish Neurotheology", CCAR Journal: The Reform Jewish Quarterly, Winter 2016.

Newberg, Andrew, and Stephanie Newberg. "A Neuropsychological Perspective on Spiritual Development." In Handbook of Spiritual Development in Childhood and Adolescence, edited by Eugene Roehlkepartain, Pamela King, Linda Wagener, and Peter Benson. London: Sage Publications, Inc., 2005

Newberg, Andrew. "The Neurotheology Link An Intersection Between Spirituality and Health", Alternative and Complimentary Therapies, Vol 21 No 1, February 2015.

Newberg, Andrew, Nancy Wintering, Dharma Khalsa, Hannah Roggenkamp, and Mark Waldman. "Meditation Effects on Cognitive Function and Cerebral Blood Flow in Subjects with Memory Loss: A Preliminary Study." Journal of Alzheimer's Disease 20, no. 2 (2010)

Nash, M. (1995), 'Glimpses of the mind', Time.

Nesse RM. Proximate and evolutionary studies of anxiety, stress and depression: synergy at the interface. Neurosci Biobehav Rev. 1999;23:895-903.

Nicolelis, Miguel. (2011) "Beyond Boundaries: The New Neuroscience of Connecting Brains with Machines---and How It Will Change Our Lives", Times Books

O'Hara, K. and Scutt, T. (1996) There is no hard problem of consciousness. Journal of Consciousness Studies 3(4), 290-302, reprinted in J. Shear (ed.) (1997) Explaining Consciousness. Cambridge, MA, MIT Press, 69-82.

Penrose, R. (1994), Shadows of the Mind (Oxford: Oxford University Press).

Penrose, R. (1989), The Emperor's New Mind: Concerning Computers, Minds and The Laws of Physics (Oxford: Oxford University Press).

Persinger, "'I would kill in God's name' role of sex, weekly church attendance, report of a religious experience and limbic lability" Perceptual and Motor Skills 1997.

Persinger "Experimental simulation of the God experience" Neurotheology 2003.

Persinger, Corradini, Clement, Keaney, et al "Neurotheology and its convergence with neuroquantology" NeuroQuantology 2010.

Persinger, Koren and St-Pierre "The electromagnetic induction of mystical and altered states within the laboratory" Journal of Consciousness Exploration and Research 2010.

Persinger "Case report: A prototypical spontaneous 'sensed presence' of a sentient being and concomitant electroencephalographic activity in the clinical laboratory" Neurocase 2008.

Persinger and Saroka "Potential production of Hughlings Jackson's "parasitic consciousness" by physiologically-patterned weak transcerebral magnetic fields: QEEG and source localization" Epilepsy & Behavior 28 (2013).

Persinger. "The neuropsychiatry of paranormal experiences". J Neuropsychiatry Clin Neurosci 2001.

Persinger. "Neuropsychological bases of god beliefs", New York: Praeger, 1987

Persinger. "Temporal lobe epileptic signs and correlative behaviors displayed by normal populations", Journal of General Psychology, 1986

Perry BD, Pollard R. Homeostasis, stress, trauma, and adaptation. A neurodevelopmental view of childhood trauma. Child Adolesc Psychiatr Clin N Am. 1998;7:33.

Puce A, Perrett D (2003) Electrophysiological and brain imaging of biological motion. Philosoph Trans Royal Soc Lond, Series B, 358: 435–445.

Ramachandran VS. Behavioral and magnetoencephalographic correlates of plasticity in the adult human brain. Proc Natl Acad Sci USA 1993; 90: 10413–20.

Ramachandran VS. Phantom limbs, neglect syndromes, repressed memories, and Freudian psychology. Int Rev Neurobiol 1994; 37: 291–333.

Ramachandran VS. Plasticity and functional recovery in neurology. Clin Med 2005; 5: 368–73.

Ramachandran VS, Hirstein W. The perception of phantom limbs. The D. O. Hebb lecture. Brain 1998; 121: 1603–30.

Ramachandran VS, Rogers-Ramachandran D, Cobb S. Touching

the phantom limb. Nature 1995; 377: 489–90.

Ramachandran VS, Rogers-Ramachandran D. Phantom limbs and neural plasticity. Arch Neurol 2000; 57: 317–20.

Ramachandran VS, Rogers-Ramachandran D. It's all done with mirrors. Sci Am Mind 2007; 18: 16–9.

Ramachandran VS, Rogers-Ramachandran D. Sensations referred to a patient's phantom arm from another subjects intact arm: perceptual correlates of mirror neurons. Med Hypotheses 2008; 70: 1233–4.

Ramachandran VS, Rogers-Ramachandran D, Stewart M. Perceptual correlates of massive cortical reorganization. Science 1992; 258: 1159–60.

Rizzolatti G, Craighero L (2004) The mirror-neuron system. Annu Rev Neurosci 27: 169–192.

Rose´n B, Lundborg G. Training with a mirror in rehabilitation of the hand. Scand J Plast Reconstr Surg Hand Surg 2005; 39: 104–8.

Roberts, TA; Smalley, J; Ahrendt, D (December 2020). "Effect of gender affirming hormones on athletic performance in transwomen and transmen: implications for sporting organisations and legislators". British Journal of Sports Medicine. 55 (11): 577–583

Rozin R Haidt J and McCauley CR (2000) Disgust. In: Lewis M, Haviland-Jones JM (eds) Handbook of Emotion. 2nd Edition. Guilford Press, New York, pp 637–653.

Saxe R, Carey S, Kanwisher N (2004) Understanding other minds: linking developmental psychology and functional neuroimaging. Annu Rev Psychol 55: 87–124.

S. J. Russell and P. Norvig, Artificial intelligence: a modern approach (3rd edition): Prentice Hall, 2009.

Smith A (1759) The theory of moral sentiments (ed. 1976). Clarendon Press, Oxford.

Schilling, Vincent. 2017, indian country today

Stein, Stephen K. 2017, The Sea in World History: Exploration, Travel, and Trade

Tesla N. "My Inventions", 1919